Certified Occupational Therapy Assistants: Opportunities and Challenges

Certified Occupational Therapy Assistants: Opportunities and Challenges

Jerry A. Johnson
Editor

Routledge
Taylor & Francis Group
New York London

Certified Occupational Therapy Assistants: Opportunities and Challenges has also been published as *Occupational Therapy and Health Care*, Volume 5, Numbers 2/3 1988.

First published by

The Haworth Press, Inc., 10 Alice Street, Binghamton, NY 13904-1580

This edition published 2013 by Routledge

711 Third Avenue, New York, NY 10017

2 Park Square, Milton Park, Abingdon, Oxon OX14 4RN

Routledge is an imprint of the Taylor & Francis Group, an informa business

LIBRARY OF CONGRESS
Library of Congress Cataloging-in-Publication Data

Certified occupational therapy assistants : opportunities and challenges / Jerry A. Johnson, editor.
p. cm.
Includes bibliographical references.
ISBN 0-86656-830-1
1. Occupational therapy – Vocational guidance. 2. Occupational therapy assistants. I. Johnson, Jerry A.
RM735.4.C47 1988
615.8'5152'024--dc19 88-11170
CIP

Certified Occupational Therapy Assistants: Opportunities and Challenges

CONTENTS

Changing of the Guard xvii

FROM THE EDITOR'S DESK 1

Career Ladder Development for Certified Occupational Therapy Assistants 7
L. Randy Strickland

Introduction 7
History of the COTA Role 8
The Evolving Role of COTAs 9
Interaction Between Assistants and Therapists 11
Model for COTA Career Ladder Development 14
Conclusion 18
Discussion 19

Supervision of the Certified Occupational Therapy Assistant: Developing a Knowledge Base and Strategy 23
Dianna Puccetti

Developing a Knowledge Base and Utilizing Existing Resources 25
Specific Supervision Strategies 28
Conclusion 33
Discussion 34

Calculating Cost Effectiveness with the Certified Occupational Therapy Assistant 37
Marilyn Dennis

Introduction 37
Overview 38
Discussion 42
Strategies for Implementation 43
Conclusion 46

Designing Job Enrichment Projects 47
Gail Lacey Clakeley

Introduction 47
Job Satisfaction 48
Job Enrichment 49
Examples of Job Enrichment Projects 51
Conclusion 52

Certified Occupational Therapy Assistants and Microcomputers 55
Barbara J. Brewer
Penni McMahon

Introduction 55
Role of the COTA 56
Microcomputers in Therapy 57
Evaluation 58
Treatment 59
Pre-Vocational Training 61
Discussion 62
Conclusion 63

Wheelchair Clinics Work 67
Jo-Ann Brant

The Wheelchair Clinic 68
The COTA's Role in the Wheelchair Clinic 69

The Interdisciplinary Team 70
Conclusion 70

Splinting Design and Fabrication in Physical Disabilities: A Splinting Assistance Program **71**
Imelda Padilla

Introduction 71
Background 72
Program Development 72
Outcomes 74
Conclusion 74
Discussion 74

The Autosyringe Backpack for Children with Cancer: A Device that Permits Mobility **77**
Debra Galvan Nordstrom

Introduction 77
Background 78
Developmental Needs of Children with Cancer 78
Occupational Therapy Goals for Pediatric Oncology Patients 79
Development of the Autosyringe Backpack 80
Conclusion 82
Discussion 83
Appendix: Backpack Construction 84

Toy Adaptations in Pediatrics **87**
Elaine Lemire

Introduction 87
Background 88
Special Project 88
Workshop 91
Discussion 91
Conclusion 92
Appendix: Instructions for Adapting Battery Operated Toys 94

Occupational Therapy and Low Vision Rehabilitation **99**
Terri L. Reichley

Low Vision and the Rehabilitation Service 100
Training with Low Vision Aids 101
Case Histories 104
Conclusion 108

The Certified Occupational Therapy Assistant as an Activity Director **111**
Alice Krawcyk

Background of the Social Adult Day Care Program 112
Purpose of the Social Adult Day Care Program 113
Admission of Clients to the Adult Day Care Program 114
Team Effort 115
The Structured Day 115
Referral Services Associated with the ADC Program 116
Role of the COTA as Activity Director 117
Conclusion 118

A Certified Occupational Therapy Assistant's Contribution to a Substance Abuse Treatment Program **119**
Karen Kunz

Introduction 119
Money Management Program 120
Exercise Program 122
Conclusion 125

Role Delineation of the Registered Occupational Therapist and the Certified Occupational Therapy Assistant in Child Psychiatry **127**
Debora A. Davidson
Babette C. Lemons

Introduction 127
Specialized Program Development 129

Supervision 131
Conclusion 131

The Roles of the Certified Occupational Therapy Assistant and the Registered Occupational Therapist in Adult Psychiatry **133**
Christine Johnson
Catherine Santos

Introduction 133
Staff Responsibilities 134
Supervision 136
Program Examples 137
Conclusion 138

Incorporating Structured Learning Therapy into Occupational Therapy Treatment of Chronic Psychiatric Patients **141**
Wendy Ellen Wallach
Daniel Hopper

Application 143
Interpersonal Skills 145
Community Interpersonal Skills 146
Abstract Interpersonal Skills 147
Discussion 147
Conclusion 148

Job Search Skills for Unemployed Psychiatric Patients **149**
Kathryn E. Wassink

Introduction 149
Background 150
Work Program: Development and Implementation 151
Case Description 1 155
Case Description 2 156
Results 157
Conclusion 157

Strategies for Resolution of Intraprofessional Conflict Related to the Role of the Certified Occupational Therapy Assistant 159
Barbara Forté

Introduction 159
Sources of Intraprofessional Conflict 160
Strategies for Conflict Resolution 165
Conclusion 167

Mysticism and Skepticism: Obstacles to the Culturalization of the Certified Occupational Therapy Assistant 169
Terry D. Brittell

Certified Occupational Therapy Assistants as a Subculture 170
Definition of Culture 171
Components of Culture 172
Barriers to COTA Involvement in Association Activities 173
Strategies for Resolution of Problems 174
Maturation of COTAs 177
Conclusion 177

Certified Occupational Therapy Assistants: Preparation for Change 181
Ronna Linroth
Penny Boulay

Introduction 181
Issues 182
Conclusion 188

Some Messages for the COTA on Image, Imagery, and Imagination 191
Phillip D. Shannon

From the Top 191
On Image 192
On Imagery 195
On Imagination 197
The Bottom Line 199

PRACTICE WATCH: THINGS TO THINK ABOUT **201**

BOOK REVIEWS

Spinal Cord Injury: A Guide to Functional Outcomes in Occupational Therapy, edited by Judy P. Hill 203
Reviewed by Michal S. Atkins

Hand Splinting, Principles and Methods (2nd Edition), by Elaine Ewing Fess and Cynthia A. Philips 205
Reviewed by Ruth Zemke

Rehabilitation Psychology Desk Reference, edited by Bruce Caplan 207
Reviewed by Cindy Burt

THOUGHTS ON LEADERSHIP . . . **211**

Certified Occupational Therapy Assistants: Reflections on Their Thirtieth Anniversary **213**
Jerry A. Johnson

ABOUT THE EDITOR

Jerry A. Johnson, MBA, EdD, OTR, FAOTA, is well known and respected as an educator, clinician, administrator, and leader in the profession of occupational therapy. She was President of the American Occupational Therapy Association for over five years, and she continues to be active professionally at local, state, and national levels. Dr. Johnson was Founder, Professor, and Director of the Occupational Therapy Program at Boston University (1963-71). More recently, she was Professor and Elias Michael Director at Washington University, Program of Occupational Therapy (1976-82). Following her tenure at Washington University, Dr. Johnson returned to clinical practice and established her own business dealing with wellness and stress management in Denver, Colorado. She is currently Editor of *Occupational Therapy in Health Care*.

Certified Occupational Therapy Assistants: Opportunities and Challenges

Changing of the Guard

Florence Cromwell has now become Editor Emerita of *Occupational Therapy in Health Care*, as the Spring issue of Volume 5, 1988, was the last issue for which she was responsible. Florence inaugurated *Occupational Therapy in Health Care* in 1984 and has, through her creative and visionary leadership and her ability to stimulate the interest of many new and prospective authors, edited 4 and 1/4th volumes.

Occupational Therapy in Health Care emerged from needs of practicing therapists for a journal that was devoted to contemporary practice. Florence perceived the needs for a journal such as this and was able to bring the idea into existence. This focus will continue as long as there is need for it. Hopefully, if new needs arise, they will also be incorporated into *Occupational Therapy in Health Care* in relevant ways.

On behalf of each of you, as authors, members of the Editorial Board, and readers, I express deep appreciation to Florence for her perceptiveness, her determination to serve and promote occupational therapists in meaningful ways, and her ongoing commitment to inform others (including professionals in other disciplines, legislators and government officials, and administrators of health agencies and organizations) about occupational therapy and the contributions that occupational therapists make to health care and to patients.

Our best wishes go with you, Florence, and with gratitude for your many contributions, we wish you success and happiness in your future endeavors.

Jerry A. Johnson
Editor

Changing of the Guard

[illegible]

FROM THE EDITOR'S DESK

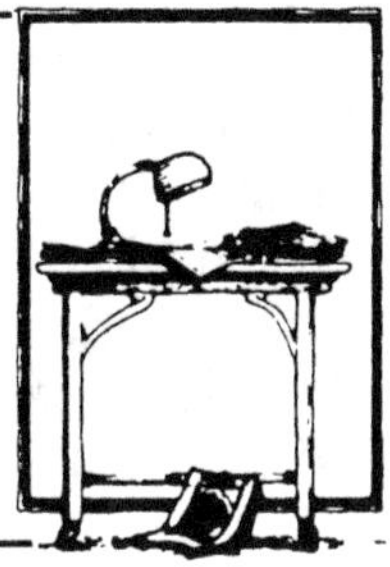

This issue is my first as the new Editor of *Occupational Therapy in Health Care*. The theme, *Certified Occupational Therapy Assistants – Challenges and Opportunities,* was selected because of its relevance to *all* occupational therapists, Occupational Therapists Registered (OTRs) and Certified Occupational Therapy Assistants (COTAs), clinicians and academicians.

Considering the history and contributions that COTAs have made to the occupational therapy profession, it is an interesting and somewhat intriguing phenomenon to observe the on-going sense of unease, and occasional conflict, that exists among occupational therapists regarding the appropriate functions and status of COTAs. There is also on-going debate about the appropriateness of allowing COTAs to fulfill certain kinds of requirements, including substitution of work experience for education, thereby enabling them to sit for the certification examination taken by graduates of professional programs at the bachelor's and master's degree levels. Successful completion of the certification examination, and its prerequisite requirements, enables individuals to use the designation Occupational Therapist Registered and to practice as occupational therapists.

The articles in this issue fall rather naturally into three categories that relate to the performance and status of COTAs and may serve as a basis for re-examination and redefinition of the relationship between occupational therapists and assistants. These categories are: (1) administrative issues regarding efficient utilization of COTAs and opportunities for career development and job satisfaction; (2) models of COTA practice described by COTAs who were responsible for developing and implementing them within the framework of their jobs; and (3) issues of concern to COTAs primarily as expressed by COTAs, with proposals and strategies for their resolution.

It is difficult to consider appropriate functions of COTAs without recognizing two of their basic contributions: cost-effectiveness and alleviation of an on-going shortage of occupational therapists which has been present in varying degrees, particularly since the post-World War II era. In fact, the education of occupational therapy assistants (or aides, as they were first named) evolved after World War II as a result of the profession's critical personnel shortage, which was compounded by the fact that there were too few occupational therapists available with appropriate academic qualifications to develop additional academic programs.

This shortage, and the successful utilization of trained technicians who assisted occupational therapists in the U.S. Army during World War II, led to the creation of job functions and educational requirement for occupational therapy assistants. Originally, occupational therapy aides, and later assistants, were perceived as being assistants to occupational therapists. However, as the practice of occupational therapy has matured and changed, as noted by several contributing authors, there have been changes in the responsibilities and functions of assistants.

Many of the authors in this issue demonstrate the ability of COTAs to be creative and productive when given specific areas or realms of responsibility for patient care. The conditions which appear to contribute to their success in program development and implementation include identification of specific patient needs by either an OTR or a COTA, sound initial planning with an OTR or other professional staff, defined areas of responsibility, good initial and on-going supervision, and willingness of COTAs to accept considerable, if not primary, responsibility for program development and implementation.

These articles demonstrate that COTAs have the potential to accept responsibility for a specific and defined area and to develop and implement programs to meet identified needs of patients and/or staff. The COTA who can develop and work in an environment which provides or requires some degree of autonomy and responsibility can be compared to technicians who work with NASA and other organizations. In these environments, the technician is one who has highly developed skills and competence in rather narrow areas, each of which contributes to a larger system or program.

Underlying the pattern of practice for COTAs described herein is the concept that occupational therapists working in this context must be both generalists and specialists. As a generalist, the occupational therapist must understand the theoretical framework which integrates all of the disparate parts into a functional system. As a specialist the occupational therapist must have knowledge, competence, and skill in programs designed for the needs of patients in a given environment. As both generalist and specialist the occupational therapist can view the system of occupational therapy practice as a matrix, have an understanding of its many dimensions, determine the system's goals and directions, exert influence on the larger system, and evaluate and modify the outcomes produced by persons working in the system.

In contrast, the occupational therapy assistant in this system acquires some in-depth expertise in one or a limited number of dimensions and may know how to transfer a given body of knowledge or set of skills from one dimension to another. It is not necessary that the assistant understand the operation of the system or know how the parts coalesce, although more experienced assistants may well acquire and utilize some of this knowledge.

The value of models such as the ones described in this issue is that they offer some very constructive possibilities for resolving some of the on-going conflicts about the appropriate functions and education of occupational therapy assistants. Another value inherent in exploration of a variety of models of practice is that they also promote examination of the appropriate levels of function and education for the occupational therapist. Every healthy system, including the practice of occupational therapy, requires the performance of a variety of levels and differing complexities of tasks.

The authors who have discussed issues of concern to COTAs in this issue have generally supported the concept of allowing COTAs to be COTAs *and* to have opportunities for advancement, recognition, and job satisfaction as COTAs, as opposed to credentialing them as OTRs. Every COTA who has the commitment to do so and is willing to make whatever sacrifices are necessary has the opportunity of applying to academic programs that prepare individuals for certification as OTRs. To be credentialed without fulfilling those requirements, both academic and clinical, negates the value of the educational process and its contributions to the professions. It also deprives the recipient of such credentialing of valuable resources that contribute to professional growth and success.

For example, at the baccalaureate degree level the importance of liberal arts as a foundation for professional education and the importance of developing a process of critical thinking are probably more widely recognized and accepted now than at any other time in American history. The contributions of liberal arts and critical thinking skills to the preparation of future occupational therapists have been documented in the 1987 document entitled *Occupational Therapy: Directions for the Future* and published by the American Occupational Therapy Association.

Perhaps the issues which should be addressed within the occupational therapy profession to resolve some of the conflicts regarding COTAs are those of (1) how best to promote and recognize the contributions of COTAs, (2) how to recognize and accept the fact that some professions need a variety of people with differing levels of education, competence, and skills, and (3) how best to provide the appropriate level of occupational therapy services to the many populations of people we serve in ways that are economical and efficient.

Differences and perceived inequality are less important and less conflictual when every individual is valued and respected for his or her individual contributions. People perceive that their contributions are of value when jobs are structured at every level to provide opportunity for growth, intellectual and emotional stimulation, rewards, and satisfaction. When all individuals within a given system know that their contributions and the contributions of others are necessary components of a healthy and functioning system, they have a sense of belonging and of shared importance.

Each COTA and each OTR contributes, in some unique way, to the successful performance of the profession in fulfilling its mission and goals. Without each of these contributions, the system would not function effectively or efficiently, and consequently, its goals would either not be met or the costs of achieving them would increase greatly.

As a profession, we have many challenges confronting us as we seek to provide services that are important to other human beings. Those challenges can lead to defeat or serve to stimulate us to act. Ultimately, it is through identification of the myriad of opportunities that are available and the selection and implementation of a select few that we move forward as a profession. The choices that occupational therapists and occupational therapy assistants make about their respective levels of education, functions and contributions may well determine the future of our profession. Hopefully, the thoughts, experiences, and beliefs of the authors who have contributed to this issue of *Occupational Therapy in Health Care* will help us make wise choices.

Jerry A. Johnson
Editor

Career Ladder Development for Certified Occupational Therapy Assistants

L. Randy Strickland, EdD, OTR, FAOTA

SUMMARY. Practice models which depict the interactions of Certified Occupational Therapy Assistants and Registered Occupational Therapists are described. These models portray career ladder development for the Certified Occupational Therapy Assistant. Job enrichment for the assistant facilitates the provision of qualitative and cost effective occupational therapy sessions.

INTRODUCTION

Certified Occupational Therapy Assistants (COTAs) currently represent a significant portion (19%) of the occupational therapy profession (American Occupational Therapy Association, 1986). From the initiation of COTA educational programs in 1958 to the present time there has been considerable discussion regarding the appropriate interaction between the therapist and the assistant (Crampton, 1958). Discussion of the conflicts between the Certified Occupational Therapy Assistant (COTA) and Registered Occupational Therapist (OTR), as well as desired practice parameters for

---

L. Randy Strickland, Director, Department of Occupational Therapy, The University of Texas Medical Branch Teaching Hospitals, Galveston, TX 77550-2777.

The author extends his appreciation to the institution's COTA and OTR staff for their exemplary role models which served as a basis for this article. Mrs. Doreen McCarty's assistance in preparing this article is gratefully appreciated.

This article appears jointly in *Certified Occupational Therapy Assistants: Opportunities and Challenges* (The Haworth Press, 1988) and *Occupational Therapy in Health Care*, Volume 5, Numbers 2/3 (1988).

each, occurred and have been reviewed at great length in various arenas for the past thirty years.

Members of the profession have continually attempted to differentiate the two levels of personnel, including education and certification requirements. These attempts have been only minimally successful in defining practice parameters for the two levels. Occupational therapy as a profession must continue to assert its place in the education and health arenas. Other forces now having an impact upon the profession also strongly suggest that clarification regarding the utilization of all occupational therapy personnel is greatly needed. For example, changing payment systems for occupational therapy services are evolving within the health care systems. Specifically, prospective payment legislation, and other fees for services have increased the emphasis upon productivity and cost effective usage of all health care personnel, including occupational therapists and assistants. Employment of COTAs provides a means of rendering cost effective quality services.

Meeting service demands can be better achieved through the development of practice models which depict COTA/OTR interaction. Examples should differentiate the different yet complementary expertise provided by the profession's two levels of personnel. Undergirding this interaction should be a developmental process promoting increased technical competency and job enrichment for the assistant. The remainder of this article provides a brief history of the COTA role and its evolution, a description of present practice with COTA/OTR interaction, and a model of a career development ladder for the assistant.

HISTORY OF THE COTA ROLE

Since 1958 the American Occupational Therapy Association (AOTA) has provided a mechanism for the formal recognition of occupational therapy assistants. Initially, COTAs underwent a training program which provided specialization in psychiatry. Graduates of COTA programs provided much needed manpower within the realm of psychiatric occupational therapy, particularly within state and federal psychiatric hospitals (Crampton, 1958).

In 1960 "AOTA Essentials of Approved Programs" were revised to provide generalized training so that assistants would be qualified to practice in varied areas of the profession (American Occupational Therapy Association, 1966). Later, two published articles described models for the utilization of the COTA. Kirchman and Howard (1966) described the role of the certified assistant in a general hospital setting as being responsible for treatment services and maintaining the supplies, equipment and the overall physical organization of the occupational therapy clinic. Adamson and Anderson (1966) discussed the utilization of occupational therapy assistants and aides in various practice settings.

Recommendations emanating from the "Entry Level Role Delineation Study" for OTRs and COTAs were developed and approved by AOTA in 1981. This study, in which entry level was defined as the first year of practice, served as a basis for establishment of standards for education and certification. The COTA was defined as an individual who works under the supervision of the OTR and may provide assistance in the evaluation, program planning and treatment processes (AOTA, 1981). Areas of independent functioning as well as the interaction between the OTR and COTA were mentioned, but no specific models were provided.

In 1985, AOTA officially adopted a paper entitled "Guide to Classification of Occupational Therapy Personnel" which recognized different work performance levels by occupational therapy assistants and therapists (AOTA, 1985). It proposed that the COTA function at three levels, including entry, intermediate, and advanced. Similar levels for the occupational therapist were also described. The "Guide" provides a possible framework for a career ladder for assistants (AOTA, 1985). This career ladder reflects the advanced clinical competency within the assistant's realm of technical responsibility.

THE EVOLVING ROLE OF COTAs

The retention and recognition of assistants is a concern for the profession, health services delivery settings and the consumer. It is important that assistants have positions with options. In Madigan's study (1985), occupational therapy assistant students identified primary career objectives as having the opportunity to (1) engage in creative pursuits and (2) specialize in a particular work area. In addition to these goals, a group of occupational therapy students also identified a desire to develop skills in research, writing, program development, and/or supervision. The difference between the occupational therapy assistant students and occupational therapy students in their career goals may prove significant in the development of the COTA/OTR team concept.

The concept of team denotes a spirit of unity within the context of a common goal. The common goal suggested in this article is the provision of quality patient services met through different, yet mutually supportive, endeavors of the therapist and assistant. The development of a collaborative relationship between the assistant and the therapist requires mutual understanding and appreciation. The goal of team cohesiveness is not attained because of the presence, or absence, of a document. Rather, creation of a team composed of a therapist and assistant requires determining which tasks are ideally performed by the assistant and are valued by the assistant. Similarly, delineated responsibilities for the occupational therapist are necessary. The occupational therapy assistant may be most interested in direct services, including the opportunity for creative pursuits in the design and delivery of program interventions.

Both the 1981 role delineation study (AOTA, 1981) and 1985 classification guide (AOTA, 1985) reflected the importance of describing the role of the COTA. Further descriptions of the utilization of occupational therapy assistants and their interactions with occupational therapists in the delivery of patient care services merit examination. The paucity in the literature of articles describing the occupational therapy assistant, and the interaction of the professional and technical levels within the profession, suggests a need to discuss and describe team building strategies for therapists and assistants. It is critical for the occupational therapy manager to be aware of such relationships. While the text *The Certified Occupational Therapy Assistant–Roles and Responsibilities* (Ryan, 1986) provides examples related to the role of the assistant, other occupational therapy texts such as *The Occupational Therapy Manager* (Bair & Gray, 1985) provide little, if any, illustrations or models regarding clinical utilization of the assistant or interactions between therapists and assistants.

There is a continuing need for additional personnel at both technical and professional levels. New and expanded arenas for occupational therapy practice can benefit from the skills of both the assistant and therapist. One way the profession will be able to truly assert its influence in the practice domain is through the successful collaboration of the therapist and the assistant and the maximum use of all manpower options.

From the perspective of cost containment, the assistant may allow for provision of treatment services with reduced financial cost to the consumer or third party payor without reduction in quality, provided there is appropriate supervision and/or consultation from the therapist. Furthermore, effective clinical utilization of the assistant's skills may provide the supervising therapist with increased opportunities for program evaluation, research, administration or other responsibilities. If cost effectiveness, including increased clinical and administrative productivity, is to become a reality, it is essential that occupational therapy personnel develop complementary practice relationships.

INTERACTION BETWEEN ASSISTANTS AND THERAPISTS

For the profession to provide the optimal health service, it is essential that effective modeling strategies utilizing both the technical and professional levels be delineated for practitioners, administrators and educators. At the University of Texas Medical Branch Teaching Hospitals in Galveston (UTMB-Galveston) a clinical practice model involving occupational therapists and assistants has existed 15 years. During this time, the institution has had opportunities to examine OTR and COTA functions and their interactions in providing patient treatment. There has been both a tradition and a calculated administrative strategy to recruit and utilize COTAs. Presently, twelve occupational therapy assistants work in a department of some sixty staff members.

The occupational therapy assistant's role should be presented as one with varied options. If the assistant aspires to provide direct care services, it is essential that this desire be translated into an action plan that provides for an orderly progression and career development track. Lippitt (1982) describes job enrichment processes as being an important means for working with the individual employee and enhancing the organization's overall productivity. By examining the role of the assistant within an agency, and considering job enrichment possibilities, it is possible to develop an individualized career plan which not only promotes the development of the employee but also the occupational therapy program, the institution, and ultimately the profession. Most importantly, a quality employee will greatly contribute to the overall delivery of excellent health services.

A critical component which supports the utilization and development of COTAs, at this institution as well as others, is a clear identification of the roles and responsibilities of assistants and therapists. Within this setting, a concerted effort has been made to define the assistant's role as involving much more responsibility than that of "assisting the therapist" or being an "extension of the therapist." Rather, the assistant's role has been developed as one which is unique within occupational therapy and which provides a viable contribution to the overall occupational therapy plan and health care plan for the patient or client.

At UTMB-Galveston the role of the occupational therapy assistant has a specialization focus. For example, it is envisioned and postulated that the assistant cannot have advanced competency in all areas of patient care. Thus, the assistant is encouraged to develop in-depth knowledge in a particular clinical or programmatic area. Consequently, the assistant develops comprehensive knowledge and skills in a particular area of practice and is able to contribute to the treatment process for those patients who require such knowledge and skills. Similarly, the occupational therapist is the individual who is charged with the overall coordination of an individual patient's program, even though the therapist may not be as skilled in particular areas of intervention services as the assistant. The therapist may serve more as a diagnostician and goal setter, though certainly using information and data provided by the assistant. The assistant may, in fact, be the individual who has the skills most needed by a particular patient or program.

The assistant's contributions are critical to the success of the treatment process. The assistant's interactions with the therapist are of a collegial nature. It is quite probable that the assistant will be providing valuable information regarding the overall development and coordination of the patient's care plan. The assistant also may be the primary treatment provider within the occupational therapy program for the patient. The therapist utilizes the special skills of the assistant and assures the coordinated attainment of treatment goals by the patient. Developing a collaborative and complementary relationship between the assistant and the therapist does not occur spontaneously. If the assistant is to develop in-depth knowledge in a particular area, it is critical that an employee development plan be implemented to achieve this result.

The therapist's role is that of the generalist who is responsible for the overall coordination of varied occupational therapy services. The assistant has the opportunity to develop skills which are highly specialized in one particular area. These contributions by the technical level of personnel within the profession allow for a more cost effective provision of patient care. Additionally, allowing the assistant to develop specialized skills within an area provides this individual with the opportunity to be more autonomous and independent in a particular area of functioning. Thus the assistant moves beyond the adjunctive role to that of a primary provider of programmatic services in varying areas of specialty.

Both levels of occupational therapy assistant staff at UTMB-Galveston are actively involved in identifying those tasks which enrich their positions. Job enrichment is a management strategy that is a serious component of any person's employment within the department. Specifically, the COTA is required to develop a special project that is conducted in addition to regularly assigned clinical duties. This special project may include areas such as program development, clinical teaching, or research. One aspect of the special project is that it be established in collaboration with the supervisor and involve interaction with the OTR or other members of the health team. Ultimately, the special project should enhance the department's mission of patient care, education, and research. Activities inherent within the special project guidelines are incorporated into the annual performance review and plan for individual employees.

Examination of the special projects undertaken by the COTAs

within this practice setting indicates that they indeed facilitate the professional development of assistants and provide a creative and appropriate interaction mechanism for the therapists and assistants. Specific examples of interaction between the therapist and assistant, as well as the use of special projects within our system, illustrate how the classification guidelines proposed by AOTA may be used in a clinical setting.

MODEL FOR COTA CAREER LADDER DEVELOPMENT

Employing occupational therapy assistants in a practice setting does not necessarily ensure effective models of professional interaction between assistants and therapists. However, throughout the history of this department, a great deal of effort has been placed upon developing collegial assistant-therapist working relationships with an ultimate goal of enhanced patient care.

One specific strategy, used with both levels of personnel within the department, has been the development of a clinical laddering system. It is important for therapists and assistants to have career ladders which allow progression from entry staff levels to advanced staff levels. Recognition of one's advanced clinical competencies and contributions to patient care may occur without requiring an individual to assume supervisory/administrative duties or acquire additional professional degrees.

The career ladder track at UTMB-Galveston is comparable to the classification system adopted by the American Occupational Therapy Association in 1985. The occupational therapist track has three levels, including Staff Occupational Therapist I (OT I), Senior Occupational Therapist (OT II), and Senior Occupational Therapist III (OT III). The Certified Occupational Therapy Assistant levels include Staff Certified Occupational Therapy Assistant (COTA I) and Senior Certified Occupational Therapy Assistant (COTA II).

Developing varied levels for COTAs may provide the foundation for the development of more collaborative relationships between the assistant and the therapist. The COTA I role serves as the entry level for the assistant. A key component of the COTA II level is the autonomy inherent in that particular role.

It is an expectation within the department that the COTA II will have advanced competencies in areas such as the design and provision of clinical programs and the ability to supervise other assistants, volunteers or selected experiences for level I occupational therapy students, among other responsibilities. Individuals who have received this professional designation, along with appropriate financial remuneration, are expected to have developed their clinical skills to performance levels providing considerable independence. While supervision may be provided on a daily basis, the individual is given a great deal of responsibility and is encouraged to exercise judgment, often in collaboration with the OTR.

Entry Level Responsibilities

A staff member who is hired as a COTA at entry level is assigned to a specific treatment team, which may or may not already have an assistant as a member. In those instances where an experienced assistant is not on the team, a concerted orientation effort is made to provide the newly hired assistant opportunities to interact with other assistants who are senior department staff members. This socialization process greatly enhances professional performance as the assistant is able to identify role models for both the assistant and therapist within the institution. This identification enables the assistant to determine parameters of practice in conjunction with the therapist.

Each assistant, regardless of classification level, is expected to be competent in the administration of patient services in the assigned area. Assigned areas for assistants are adult, child, adolescent psychiatry; adult physical rehabilitation; acute physical disabilities; geriatrics; and acute and rehabilitation pediatrics. Additionally, assistants have been used in home health programs. Regardless of assignment area, the entry level assistant is oriented to the roles of other assistants within the department, as well as being provided orientation to one's own particular job duties on the specific team.

To illustrate assignments for assistants, the rehabilitation program uses an entry level assistant to provide personal daily living skills training for patients during the morning. The assistant provides patient education and carries out treatment regimes established by the therapist such as cognitive training and self-care tasks.

It is also possible for this assistant to develop independent programming skills through several options which are required on this unit. For instance, the COTA conducts an evening program which stresses the patient's attainment of ADL skills required for community reintegration and independent living. The assistant is charged with the responsibility of independently planning and implementing this weekly activity. This work task requires interaction and planning with other members of the health team. While general supervision is received from the therapist, it is the assistant's responsibility to determine the focus of the activity and how the activity must be adapted to the needs of particular patients. This provides an opportunity of independent problem solving on a specific assignment while still receiving other more structured treatment assignments.

It is important to note that in this example there is a balance of clinical activities requiring different levels of autonomy. It has been demonstrated clinically, in this particular unit, that a balance between structured treatment assignments and those which allow greater creativity require the assistant to broaden the professional skills for program planning and to be a more active participant in the overall treatment process.

Intermediate Level Responsibilities

After working within a practice setting for at least a year, the assistant is considered to be experienced (and beyond entry level) if the work requirements set forth in the initial performance plan have been met. Assistants may advance into the COTA II level or continue to be designated as COTA I's. The assistant who has met job performance expectations is provided with additional responsibilities and opportunities for professional growth. Supervision of the COTA by either an experienced OTR or COTA is more general in nature and not as specifically focused as that provided to entry level assistants.

One example of an individual's successful functioning at this level involves staff members assigned to adult psychiatry. Within this program, both occupational therapists and occupational therapy assistants provide evaluation and treatment services. The certified assistant on this particular team assists with evaluation and is an important member of the team in obtaining evaluative data regarding patient performance. In acute psychiatry functional assessment and appropriate community program recommendations from occupational therapy are critical functions. The assistant in this setting administers daily living skills evaluations such as meal preparation and budgeting areas, provides structured tasks to evaluate cognitive performance and reports patient performance on such activities. This assistant may provide supervision for occupational therapy assistant students, participate in the inservice program and contribute to program development through presentations.

Another intermediate level COTA staff member has been very successful in participating in a collaborative relationship with the OTR in the provision of geriatric rehabilitation services. This assistant is responsible for the development of daily activity groups for geriatric patients as well as provision of individual self-care training programs for patients.

While the occupational therapist on the geriatric rehabilitation unit is responsible for patient assessment, evaluation data is obtained and recorded by the assistant. Similarly, while specialized neuromuscular rehabilitation techniques and protocols are initially implemented by the therapist, they are often later reinforced by the assistant with general supervision from the OTR. The two individuals jointly plan the treatment regime for individual patients and depending upon unit needs, provide instruction to staff and family members regarding patient progress and future needs.

Advanced Level Responsibilities

Our career development planning model uses a process providing focused task specific supervision for the entry level assistant. With increased technical competency in a specific practice arena, the COTA may assume greater responsibility for program planning and implementation and be recognized as a senior staff member (COTA II). As a result of such program development, assistants from the department have made clinical presentations at both state and national conferences regarding the programs developed in collaboration with OTRs. Other assistants have been involved in projects which describe their programs or activities through case examples or written articles. Assistants at UTMB-Galveston are not a second tier level of staff but participate as full members of the health team.

For example, one COTA within the department has developed a

great deal of expertise in the area of adaptive equipment. The assistant has become very skilled at the utilization of switches and technological aids for the adaptation of toys for children with severely limiting physical conditions. This COTA has developed an instruction manual for use with public school districts and other community agencies and has independently provided workshops regarding toy adaptation for children. Furthermore, she regularly teaches toy adaptation to agency staff and students. All these activities are performed with consultation from the supervising OTR. On occasion, she and the supervising OTR have jointly designed adaptive toy items. This, again, is another example of a special enrichment project that has encouraged an individual to go far beyond the parameters that might have originally been envisioned in the area of adaptive equipment.

A work preparation program developed by another assistant prepares psychiatric patients to re-enter the work force by using an instructional package and program which presents the basics of preparing to re-enter the job market. The COTA determines with the supervising OTR which patients should enter the program. The OTR monitors patient progress while the actual instruction and design of patient programs is the responsibility of the COTA. The success of this program is demonstrated by the feedback from patients who have indeed successfully returned to the community. Unsolicited letters and telephone calls of praise have been received from community counselors.

CONCLUSION

Occupational therapy assistants at UTMB-Galveston have the opportunity and responsibility to develop special projects or programs. They often have developed these projects in coordination with and consultation with supervising OTRs. While the ultimate responsibility for the assessment and the treatment of the patient rests with the therapist, our career ladder focus promotes the development of working conditions which facilitate each individual assistant's performance and ability to creatively pursue career goals.

Assistants throughout the department have staff assignments and projects reflective of varying competency levels. This differs from those settings in which the assistant's role has been that of assisting the therapist. In this department both assistants and therapists assist the patient. Consequently, we promote a philosophy that allows staff members to develop programs utilizing advanced expertise, to collaborate with other department staff and members of the health team, and most importantly to communicate with patients regarding the aims and focus of specific occupational therapy programs.

Assistants provided with opportunities to develop and offer programs appear to have a greater investment in the program, and many assistants have been with the department for five to seven years. We continue recruiting new assistants to the program and believe that our job enrichment strategies offer a significant recruiting and retention advantage. Additionally, the COTA does assist in maintaining a more reasonable cost structure for the provision of occupational therapy services. Provision of billable patient services and high productivity levels by the COTA allows increased OTR emphasis on program development, education and clinical research. Through careful training and the development of our assistants we have been able to develop a treatment model which is cost effective and qualitative.

While assistants tend to specialize within specific clinical areas, such specialization does not necessarily inhibit the assistant's performance in other areas if reassignment to different practice settings is required. Developed expertise in an area of occupational therapy should be transferable to numerous other settings within the department or within other practice settings provided the individual has learned the process of transferring knowledge or skills. The department has experienced numerous benefits as a result of the activities of its assistants. As previously described, special programs have received praise from individuals both within and outside the institution because of the efforts of our assistants.

DISCUSSION

This article has described the philosophy and operational plan for developing a career ladder for occupational therapy assistants. Using the "Guide to the Classification of Occupational Therapy Personnel" (AOTA, 1985) as a frame of reference, it is possible for members of occupational therapy programs to develop different levels of performance expectations for occupational therapy assistants and therapists. Through the use of such a guide or similar process, it is possible to assure provision of quality occupational therapy services and promote the development of occupational therapy personnel. Descriptions of occupational therapy assistants' functions in various position levels discussed in the AOTA classification guide may be useful to other therapists and assistants developing practice models. While the models described in this article are possible examples of COTA roles, perhaps they will stimulate more discussion and development of new possibilities for COTAs.

It seems appropriate to note that Certified Occupational Therapy Assistants, a personnel category formally recognized in 1958, are now approaching the magical age of thirty. Sheehy (1974) describes the developmental stage of one's twenties as being that of trying and testing, while the thirties are a time to make new choices and commitments. Careful examination of effective utilization of assistants will facilitate interaction between the COTA and the OTR and will lead to the probability that assistants will have a more profound and marked influence upon the provision of occupational therapy services during the next decade.

With continuation of personnel shortages and the need to be cost effective, internal recognition of the two staff levels is an economic reality. By effectively utilizing COTAs, the profession may be able to better exert its influence within the health arena and more positively and appropriately enhance the overall provision of quality patient care through occupational therapy services. The COTA's role has been ill-defined in the past, but it is now time to recognize the important contributions that have and can be made by assistants and to develop strategies which enhance assistant/therapist interactions and the career development for both levels of occupational therapy personnel.

REFERENCES

Adamson, M. J., & Anderson, M. A. (1966). Study of the utilization of occupational therapy assistants and aides. *American Journal of Occupational Therapy, 20*, 75-79.

American Occupational Therapy Association (1966). Board of management: Mid-year meeting reports. *American Journal of Occupational Therapy, 14*, 232.

American Occupational Therapy Association (1981). *Entry level role delineation for OTRs and COTAs*. (No. VII.1-VII.10). Rockville, MD: American Occupational Therapy Association, Inc.

American Occupational Therapy Association (1985). Guide to classification of occupational therapy personnel. *American Journal of Occupational Therapy, 39*, 803-810.

American Occupational Therapy Association (1986). *1986 member data survey*. Rockville, MD: American Occupational Therapy Association, Inc.

Bair, J., & Gray, M. (1985). *The occupational therapy manager*. Rockville, MD: American Occupational Therapy Association, Inc.

Crampton, M. W. (1958). The recognition of occupational therapy assistants. *American Journal of Occupational Therapy, 12*, 269-275.

Kirchman, M. M., & Howard, B. (1966). Role of the certified assistant in a general hospital. *American Journal of Occupational Therapy, 20*, 293-297.

Lippitt, G. L. (1982). *Occupational renewal* (2nd edition). Englewood Cliffs, NJ: Prentice-Hall, Inc.

Madigan, M. J. (1985). Characteristics of students in occupational therapy educational programs. *American Journal of Occupational Therapy, 39*, 41-48.

Ryan, S. E. (1986). *The certified occupational therapy assistant–roles and responsibilities*. Thorofare, NJ: Slack, Inc.

Schwagmeyer, M. (1969). The certified occupational therapy assistant today. *American Journal of Occupational Therapy, 23*, 69-70.

Sheehy, G. (1974). *Predictable crises of adult life*. New York: E. P. Dutton.

Supervision of the Certified Occupational Therapy Assistant: Developing a Knowledge Base and Strategy

Dianna Puccetti, OTR

SUMMARY. As current trends in health care continue to develop, manpower demands within the profession of occupational therapy will continue to rise. Creative partnerships and collaborative efforts between therapists and assistants are rapidly becoming a necessity to provide cost-effective patient care within a variety of treatment settings. Several documents and resources concerning role delineation and supervision of assistants are available within the literature; however, few resources have been compiled to address supervision and supervision strategies for the assistant.

This paper addresses supervision of the assistant in a fairly broad and generic sense, and includes specific strategies that may be introduced to enhance the supervisory process.

Effective supervision and strategies for management of staff are critical components of any working relationship. Efficient management of staff to meet the ever increasing demands of the health care system is perhaps one of the biggest challenges facing the occupational therapy supervisor of today and of the future (Occupational Therapy Newspaper, 1984). As registered occupational therapists

---

Dianna Puccetti, Occupational Therapist III, Physical Disabilities Division, Occupational Therapy Department, University of Texas Medical Branch Teaching Hospitals, Galveston, TX 77550.

This article appears jointly in *Certified Occupational Therapy Assistants: Opportunities and Challenges* (The Haworth Press, 1988) and *Occupational Therapy in Health Care*, Volume 5, Numbers 2/3 (1988).

(therapists) address these demands, effective use of certified occupational therapy assistants (assistants) will become increasingly important in providing cost-effective services. Several documents exist in the literature that describe role delineation, mobility or career opportunities, and supervision of assistants. However, to date, there are few publications that address utilization of existing information and its application to supervision of assistants.

Ambiguity exists in relation to supervision of the assistant and presents a dilemma both for the supervising therapist and the assistant. It is at times difficult to assess exactly when and how to enter into the supervisory process. It is equally difficult to know when to remain silent or to simply monitor the assistant's performance. To some extent, an effective supervisor needs to have an intuitive sense that complements specific supervision strategies. An analogy which illustrates this perspective occurred while preparing this article. As I was leaving our administrative offices presently located in temporary quarters during hospital renovation, I noted a construction worker's sign scrawled and propped against the wall which read:

CONSTRUCTION AREA
DO NOT ENTER
DANGER – WORK

Being preoccupied with the task of formulating this paper, the sign's message transferred immediately to the tasks of supervision. There are, of course, obvious differences between the concrete task of constructing walls and ceilings, and the sometimes concrete, but most often, more abstract task of supervising staff. Supervision of staff could certainly be equated with the concept of a "construction area." Supervisors are, in fact, assisting with "constructing" the development of their staff. But, the following words on the construction worker's sign *DO NOT ENTER* do not support the concept of supervision at all. Supervision is an area in which supervisors want to be "actively" involved and engaged in on a daily basis; and while the last words, *DANGER – WORK* are in fact true, supervision *is* work, but it is work that can be very gratifying and productive.

When addressing the topic of supervision, and specifically related it to the assistant, three concerns merit review. First, an effective supervisor needs to have a clear understanding of the role of the assistant, both at entry-level and as the assistant gains experience. Second, supervision need to be tailored to "individual" needs and styles. Last, and perhaps most critical, the supervisor is one of the primary people to offer job enhancement *and* personal growth to assistants under their direction.

It is essential that the supervisor and the assistant have a reciprocal understanding of each other's styles of interaction to establish and maintain open communication. It is also imperative that the supervisor and assistant assume certain responsibilities in the supervisory process. The supervisor is responsible for helping the assistant to identify personal and professional needs and to define necessary or desired directions within the program setting. The supervisor also promotes a climate which allows the assistant to gain acceptance and approval for implementation of new ideas. Within this process, the assistant is responsible to remain open and accepting of supervision and collaboration (Blechert & Christensen, 1986).

Through the development of this paper, a clear understanding of supervision of the assistant utilizing existing resources will emerge. Supervision will be defined, suggested and mandated supervision requirements will be discussed, information on role delineation will be presented and psychological expectations of supervision will be addressed. In addition, specific strategies designed to enhance and guide supervision will be presented.

DEVELOPING A KNOWLEDGE BASE AND UTILIZING EXISTING RESOURCES

Definition of Supervision

According to *Webster's New World Dictionary* (1974), the term "supervise" is defined as follows: "to oversee; direct, or manage; superintend." The word supervision can also be less formally defined as the process by which work or workers are directed and managed. This definition supports the idea that the supervisor is a primary or key person to provide direction, job enhancement and personal growth for the supervisee or assistant. *The American Occupational Therapy Association (AOTA) Official Position Paper on Supervision* gives further credence to this concept (AOTA, 1981).

Suggested Supervisory Standards

Specific guidelines which govern supervision of the assistant can be found in the AOTA resource, "Guide to Classification of Occupational Therapy Personnel" (AOTA, 1985). This document outlines work performance definitions for all levels of occupational therapy staff, including the assistant. It also includes directives for entry-level, intermediate, and advanced staff. Critical performance areas are listed as clear and well defined statements describing the supervisory support needed at each level of performance.

Entry-Level Role Delineations

An additional AOTA resource, "Entry Level Role Delineation of OTRS and COTAs," is available to define the role delineation and the supervision needs of the assistant (AOTA, 1981). In 1981, AOTA adopted entry-level role delineations for therapists and assistants, and to date, the statements contained in this document have served to define roles and to clarify necessary skills for the entry-level therapist and assistant. The role delineation statements also serve to assist in the development of educational essentials. The original document included the following categories: referral, occupational therapy assessment, program planning, occupational therapy treatment, program discontinuation, service management, continued education and public relations. Knowledge and understanding of these entry-level guidelines is critical for the assistant's supervisor. Successful interaction between the supervisor and assistant requires a thorough understanding of these guidelines.

Most recently, in 1986, AOTA initiated a Professional and Technical Role Analysis Project (PATRA) which examined existing role assignments for both entry-level assistants and therapists during the first year of practice. Critical components of the PATRA project include the identification of task statements reflecting current practice, and the knowledge, skills and attitudes essential for task mastery. A final project report is scheduled for presentation to the 1988 Representative Assembly (*Occupational Therapy News*, 1987).

AOTA resources have provided useful and general guidelines for supervision of assistants at various stages of their professional development. Application of these guidelines can provide an avenue for feedback that offers varying amounts of supervision to meet the needs of the individual assistant.

In those states with licensure laws, therapists are required to follow the state statutes relative to supervision of assistants. These rules may vary from state to state, and it is the responsibility of the supervisor to remain knowledgeable in their interpretation and application.

Psychological Expectations of Supervision

Another valuable resource that offers information on supervision of the assistant is *The Certified Occupational Therapy Assistant–Roles and Responsibilities* (Ryan, 1986). There, supervision of the assistant is described in terms of a socialization process or metamorphosis which begins with academic preparation and continues and builds through fieldwork experiences, then on to entry-level work experiences, self-enhancement activities and finally to the level of the socialized assistant who has mastered the level of an advanced technical clinician and whose commitment to the profession is evident. Within this text, supervision of the assistant and practical applications of supervisory theory are presented.

Many of the concepts in Ryan's book are derived from the work of Levinson, a clinical psychologist, who in 1962 developed the idea of a "psychological contract" between an individual and the work place. Levinson described certain *needs* that each person has in relation to the work place (Levinson, 1962). These needs are described by the three terms *ministration, mastery* and *maturation*. Definitions of each of these terms or needs clearly correlate with supervision needs. *Ministration* needs relate to a desire to feel close to others in the work setting and the desire for support, guidance and protection. *Mastery* is the need to explore, to understand and to exercise some control over oneself and the environment. *Matura-*

tion needs define the desire for feedback and growth experiences to attain an advanced level of skill.

Application of Levinson's definitions of needs support and guide the assistant through this psychological process. When these needs are met, there are some specific outcomes for the worker and supervisor including a respectful working relationship, a productive work environment, the ability to manage stress in a constructive manner, and the ability to recognize individual strengths and weaknesses to maximize work performance. If all these psychological needs are fulfilled, an individual develops on a professional level, and if they are not fulfilled, the person stagnates, and negative consequences occur.

SPECIFIC SUPERVISION STRATEGIES

Thus far this presentation has focused on the formal definition of supervision, suggested and mandated supervision requirements, and role delineation and psychological expectations of supervision. More specific strategies and their applications in the work place will now be considered.

The following supervision strategies and tools have been used successfully in supervision of therapists and assistants within the Physical Disabilities Division at the University of Texas Medical Branch Hospitals. These tools are valuable and easy to use and could easily be adapted for other settings. Tools to be described include: The New Therapist Questionnaire/Checklist (Figure 1), the Career Planning and Assessment Form (Figure 2), and the Special Project Form (Figure 3). The forms to be described help to facilitate supervision with staff, but more importantly, these forms help to structure the daily interaction between the staff member and the supervisor. They offer direct feedback that includes validation of a job well done or constructive criticism and problem solving directives in areas that require improved performance.

New Therapist Questionnaire/Checklist

The New Therapist Questionnaire/Checklist was developed in 1985 by a task force committee within the Physical Disabilities Division at UTMB. When a new therapist or assistant is hired or when an employee transfers into the Physical Disabilities Division, the New Therapist Questionnaire/Checklist (Figure 1) is introduced to that staff member. The form is generally completed during the first week of employment. Each therapist follows an instruction sheet to complete his or her form. By completing the form, staff members can clearly rate their existing knowledge and skill based on previous education and work experience. This information, in turn, is uti-

INSTRUCTIONS FOR THE NEW THERAPIST QUESTIONNAIRE/CHECKLIST

During your first week of work, complete the first column of the questionnaire using the provided key.

In the months of your probationary period, you will be given opportunities to increase your knowledge/proficiency in areas appropriate to your team and areas of particular interest to you.

This form will be used as a guideline for you and your supervisor and will document efforts made to increase your proficiency.

Your supervisor will rate the items on the checklist according to the priorities of your team:

2 - Indicates high priority; should be mastered by your 2 month performance report

4 - Indicates middle priority; should be mastered by your 4 month performance report

6 - Indicates lower priority; should be mastered by 6 month performance report

Those areas not rated 2, 3 or 6 will be considered areas in which proficiency is not necessary for your team and which can be pursued as areas of interest if desired.

In the follow-up column, you and your supervisor will document level of experience for pertinent items using the following key:

O -- Observed. You observed this item performed by another therapist. Dated.

A -- Assisted. You assisted in this item but did not initiate or perform independently. Dated.

P -- Performed. You performed independently. Dated.

P.O. -- Performed independently and observed by supervisor or another therapist.

Other comments may be included in this column: pertinent reading, lectures, tapes, workshops, etc.

Note: For those items which are a high priority for your team, your supervisor will probably want to observe your performance, regardless of initial level of experience.

FIGURE 1

UTMB SAMPLE OCCUPATIONAL THERAPY NEW THERAPIST
QUESTIONNAIRE/CHECKLIST

Key: 1 = Have not had experience with
2 = Observed (or classroom instruction)
3 = Participated in under supervision
4 = Participated in without supervision

* = Star areas that are of special interest to you

A. Evaluations		Follow-up
1. ROM - goniometry - passive		
2. ROM - functional		
3. MMT - specific		
4. MMT - gross, functional		
5. Grip Strength - Dynamometer		
6. Sensory		
a. 2 point - classic		
b. sharp-dull		
c. light touch		
d. vibration		
e. moving touch		
f. moving 2 pt.		
g. Tinel's sign		
h. Phalen's sign		
i. temperature		
j. proprioception		
k. stereognosis		
l. graphesthesia		
m. Moberg pick up test		
n. hypersensitivity		
o. skin wrinkling		

FIGURE 1 (continued)

lized by the staff member and supervisor to plan experiences to increase knowledge, skill and proficiency in areas appropriate to assigned teams and individual interests.

The New Therapist Questionnaire/Checklist is divided into the following categories: (A) Evaluation, (B) Treatment for Specific Diagnoses, and (C) Treatment Techniques. Within each of these categories are very specific items which relate to evaluation, treatment techniques or skills. Staff rate each item according to the printed key. Once the form is completed, the supervisor and staff member discuss the information and collaboratively rate the items on the checklist and establish priorities for the assigned area. Numbers 2, 4 and 6 are used by the supervisor to designate skills and/or proficiencies to be attained on any particular item at the two, four, or six month period during the staff member's probation. The form is then used during supervisory sessions and probationary performance reports to document proficiency or acquisition of new skills and knowledge.

Career Planning and Assessment Form

Another useful tool is the Career Planning and Assessment Form (Figure 2). This form was developed to encourage staff to examine their job roles and skills, and it encourages therapists and assistants to assume an active role and responsibility for planning professional development. Prior to the scheduled evaluation date, the supervisor and the staff member being evaluated complete the form separately. At the time of the performance evaluation, forms are exchanged. If the supervisor is in tune with the staff member, there should be a validating exchange of information. If obvious differences occur, the written statements serve to initiate discussion concerning the points in question.

Special Project Form

An additional form is the Special Project Form (Figure 3). Each staff member is required to be involved in at least one special project, usually designed by the individual staff member during the year. The form is used to provide guidance to a staff member when planning a project. It also provides a mechanism for problem solving through the outline of project steps and process. Projects are not initiated until after the six month probationary period is complete and must be approved by the staff member's direct-line supervisor, the Assistant Director of the Division, and/or the Director of the Department prior to implementation.

Another important framework for supervision that cannot be overemphasized in importance is the weekly or biweekly individual supervision session. These sessions can vary in length and can be used to discuss issues that may be facing the staff member. They also provide a structured mechanism to discuss strengths, limitations, goals and needs. Very often these sessions are used for planning new activities or goals and the expected time lines for completion of any proposed activity. It is generally helpful for the supervisor to maintain a written record of agenda items discussed as a reference. This record can be kept in a variety of ways such as an informal handwritten log, or in a more formal manner, by typed

Figure 2

CAREER PLANNING AND ASSESSMENT

Staff: ______________________

Key tasks

List your major areas of responsibility or key tasks in your job.

Obstacles

Were there any obstacles which hindered you from accomplishing what you would have wished? Are they likely to recur?

Past year's work

What have you done best or with greatest satisfaction?

Improvement

To make your job performance better, what changes might be made by:

a. Your immediate supervisor or higher management?

b. Yourself?

c. Anyone else?

Career

What are your goals for the coming year?

What continuing education experiences would you like to pursue?

What continuing education experiences have you attended over the past year?

What do you feel are your strengths and weaknesses?

Additional Comments:

minutes of the session. It is important that a supervisor develop a method and style that is meaningful and comfortable for that individual.

In addition to utilizing the forms described above, the Department has developed Uniform Job Descriptions for all levels of staff. These job descriptions help improve employee performance by clar-

Figure 3

PERFORMANCE EVALUATIONS

SPECIAL PROJECT

1. What topic have your chosen for your project?

2. Why or how do you think this project will benefit you, others, realm of occupational therapy?

3. Who other than yourself will you need support from (others in dept., other disciplines)?

4. What materials, finances will you need to complete this activity?

5. When would you be able to initiate this project?

6. What could be accomplished in the first 6 months?

7. How long would it take to complete this project?

8. How frequently would you like to meet with the Assistant Director to receive assistance, support, etc.?

9. Is this a project in which the data could be published, presented as an inservice to dept., district, state, national meeting?

ifying expectations and by providing a very objective tool on which to base an employee's performance and evaluation.

CONCLUSION

The resources, ideas and strategies contained in this paper are intended to assist therapists in strengthening their understanding of the supervisory needs of the assistant. While the present knowledge base regarding supervision of the assistant has been considered, many areas of question remain. For example, this author discusses supervision of the assistant but does not address the need for specific determination of assistant competencies in performance of professional tasks. The question then needs to be stated: What are the specific tasks and competencies appropriate for the assistant? Delineating those tasks which appropriately remain within the practice parameters of the assistant is a complex task filled with ambiguity for the supervisor and assistant. The profession may, in the future, consider the development of a practice hierarchy which would strengthen clarification of practice roles and address supervisory relationships in more explicit terms.

DISCUSSION

This author has combined existing resources and data with specific supervisory strategies that have been used successfully. In reconsidering the "construction zone" analogy a careful case has been made for developing a "supervisory blueprint." This blueprint, drawn from guidelines, role delineations, and supervisory methods, establishes a foundation for effective supervision of the assistant.

Guides exist within the literature which suggest supervision strategies for the assistant. Using available information as building blocks, a supervisory approach for assistants has been developed and based upon an open communication process between the supervisor and staff member. This process is strengthened by mutual understanding and acceptance of individual differences, strengths and needs.

The specific strategies outlined have offered further support of an ongoing and open supervisory system designed specifically to promote employee growth and development. Particular emphasis has been placed on the orientation and training program for the assistant utilizing a structured approach. Additional critical components, including career planning and development have been identified and expanded. Undergirding all of these strategies is ongoing dialogue and counseling between the supervisor and assistant.

Hopefully, this article has presented a starting point for the development of expanded supervisory models for assistants. The compilation of resources including existing data and specific strategies used in one clinical facility represents a beginning step. It is now necessary to further define and develop this topic to effectively respond to the ever increasing demands of the health care system and the needs of our profession.

REFERENCES

American Occupational Therapy Association (1981). *Entry level role delineation for OTRs and COTAs*. (Reference Manual of the Official Documents of the American Occupational Therapy Association, Inc., VII.1-VII.10). Rockville, MD.

American Occupational Therapy Association (1985). Guide to classification of occupational therapy personnel. *American Journal of Occupational Therapy, 39*, 803-810.

American Occupational Therapy Association (1981). Guide for supervision of occupational therapy personnel. *American Journal of Occupational Therapy, 35*, 815-816.

American Occupational Therapy Association (1984). OT among twenty fastest growing occupations. *Occupational Therapy Newspaper, 33*:3, p. 6.

Blechert, T.F. & Christensen, M.F. (1986). Intraprofessional relationships and socialization: The maturation process. In S.E. Ryan (Ed.), *The certified occupational therapy assistant–roles and responsibilities*, pp. 377-390. Thorofare, NJ: Slack, Inc.

Guralnik, D.B. (Ed.) (1974). *Webster's new world dictionary*, Second College Edition, p. 1430. New York: William Collins & World Publishing Co., Inc.

Levinson, H. (1962). *Men, management, and mental health*. Cambridge, MA: Harvard University Press.

Ryan, S.E. (1986). *The certified occupational therapy assistant–roles and responsibilities*. Thorofare, NJ: Slack, Inc.

Spelbring, L. (1987). PATRA project final activity underway. *Occupational Therapy News, 41*:8, p. 5.

Calculating Cost Effectiveness with the Certified Occupational Therapy Assistant

Marilyn Dennis, MPA, OTR

SUMMARY. The need for occupational therapists continues to rise during a time when those in health care management must also concern themselves with containing costs. This paper compares the expense of an all therapist department vs. a department comprised of therapists and assistants. Appropriate assignment of therapists vs. assistants in various clinical settings is discussed. The paper also describes how one multiclinic department redefined two assistant positions to enhance productivity.

INTRODUCTION

Bonnie Brooks (1982) encouraged members of the American Occupational Therapy Association to be concerned not only with the internal issues effecting the Certified Occupational Therapy Assistant, but also with external issues and their impact upon the occupational therapy profession. She wrote,

> With limited numbers of professionals available to meet the increase in demand for services, members must individually and collectively develop innovative strategies to deal with the constantly expanding role of occupational therapy. Role models

---

Marilyn Dennis is Assistant Director in the Occupational Therapy Department at the University of Texas Medical Branch, Galveston, TX. She received her Occupational Therapy Degree from the University of Kansas and her master's degree in Public Administration from the University of Missouri at Kansas City.

This article appears jointly in *Certified Occupational Therapy Assistants: Opportunities and Challenges* (The Haworth Press, 1988) and *Occupational Therapy in Health Care*, Volume 5, Numbers 2/3 (1988).

> and studies are needed to clearly demonstrate that Registered Occupational Therapists (therapist) working effectively with Certified Occupational Therapy Assistants (assistant) in a unified effort results in an expansion of occupational therapy services and is cost effective as well. (Brooks, 1982, p. 568)

Five years later this demand for therapists has escalated. Projections for the future suggest that the demand for occupational therapy services should increase well into the year 2050 (Manpower Commission Report, AOTA, 1986).

OVERVIEW

Several practice models are available describing the working relationship of the therapist and assistant (*Occupational Therapy News*, 1987; Strickland, 1988). Although quality of care, positive working relationships, and expansion of occupational therapy services are desirable outcomes, the *cost savings* of these practice strategies is often the selling point in presenting such staffing patterns to hospital administrators.

Information from the *1986 Member Data Survey* (AOTA, 1987) indicated the mean income for the full-time employed Registered Occupational Therapist was $26,528 while the mean for the full-time employed Certified Occupational Therapy Assistant was $16,182. Although the mean salaries for both the therapist and assistant may continue to change, the variance between the two probably remains relatively the same; thus, a salary savings of approximately $10,000 can be realized when hiring an assistant rather than a therapist.

By utilizing some simple accounting principles, it is possible to compare the cost savings of an occupational therapy department comprised of all therapists versus one consisting of therapists and assistants. To determine departmental expenses, the occupational therapy manager must calculate both direct and indirect expenses. At the University of Texas Medical Branch (UTMB), *direct expenses* are costs directly related to the operation of the department and include all departmental staff salaries, service contracts, supplies and equipment. *Indirect expenses* are those costs indirectly related to the operation of the department and include building depreciation, employee health and welfare, administrative services, physical plant, laundry and housekeeping. Indirect expenses are charged to departmental budgets on a formula, often based on square footage of the department. At UTMB indirect expenses are computed as 75% of the total projected direct expenses.

Consider a ten member department consisting of ten therapists versus a department of five therapists and five assistants. If one generates direct expense costs for salaries based on the 1986 membership survey data, the mean annual income of the therapist and assistant can be calculated. Table 1 illustrates the total salary costs of the two departments. The ten therapist department, Department

Table 1

A Comparison of the Total Salary Cost of an Occupational Therapy Department Comprised of all Therapists Versus a Department Comprised of Therapists and Assistants[1]

	POSITION	ANNUAL SALARY[2]	STAFF	TOTAL SALARY COST[3]
Department One	OTR	$26,528	10	$265,280
Department Two	OTR	$26,528	5	$132,640
	COTA	16,182	5	80,910
				$213,550

[1]The above comparison does not suggest that all OTR staffed hospitals could function under the COTA/OTR ratio described in Department #2. Instead, the comparison illustrates only the statistical techniques available for realizing the cost savings of staffing COTAs and OTRs.

[2]Annual Salary based on 1986 AOTA Member Data Survey

[3]Total Salary Cost should also include salaries of administrative and support staff and fringe benefits of all staff. These items were not figured in to maintain simplicity of calculations.

One, has a total salary cost of $265,280. Department Two, consisting of five therapists and five assistants, has a total salary cost of $213,550, which is a savings of $51,730 for Department Two.

Service contracts, supplies, and equipment are also a portion of the direct expense. These costs are apt to be the same for both departments. A $40,000 cost is suggested for these items and is added to the salary cost for both departments to obtain a more realistic total for projected direct expense. Table 2 outlines these statistics. The total direct expense, then, for Department One becomes $305,280 while the total direct expense for Department Two is $253,550.

If a facility defines indirect expense as a percentage of the direct expense then the department would realize an additional cost savings if assistants had been hired rather than therapists. As stated earlier, UTMB calculates indirect expense as 75% of direct expense. The total projected costs are defined as direct plus indirect expense. These calculations are shown in Table 3. The total projected cost for Department One is estimated as being $534,240 while the total projected cost for Department Two is $443,712. The cost savings to a facility which has hired the five therapists and five assistants as compared to the ten therapist department is $90,258 (see Table 3).

If the market in which you work is highly competitive, this cost

Table 2

A Comparison of the Total Direct Expense of an Occupational Therapy Department Comprised of all Therapists Versus a Department Comprised of Therapists and Assistants.

	TOTAL SALARY COST	+ MAINTENANCE & OPERATIONS	= TOTAL PROJECTED DIRECT EXPENSE
Department One	$265,280	$40,000	$305,280
Department Two	213,550	40,000	253,550

Table 3

A Comparison of the Total Projected Cost of an Occupational Therapy Department Comprised of all Therapists Versus a Department Comprised of Therapists and Assistants.

	TOTAL PROJECTED DIRECT EXPENSE	+	INDIRECT EXPENSE	=	TOTAL PROJECTED COST
Department One	$305,280		75% X $305,280		$534,240
Department Two	253,550		75% X 253,550		443,712
					$ 90,528 (Difference in Total Projected Cost between Depart- One and Two)

UTMB Indirect expense equals 75% of Direct Expense and Includes building depreciation, employee health & welfare, administrative services, physical plant, laundry, housekeeping. Various formulas are used in determining indirect expense. This is the formula used by UTMB Hospital Accounting.

savings could be passed on to the consumer, otherwise known as the patient or 3rd party payor, whichever the case may be. To describe this savings most simply, it is suggested that the two departments being compared are self-sufficient, not for profit. Both departments' productivity standards require a daily average of 18 chargeable units of 15 minutes per therapist. There are 249 working days in a year (exclusive of Saturdays, Sundays, and holidays), and each staff member receives two weeks of vacation. It is anticipated that each staff member will use an average of five sick and administrative days per year suggesting that each therapist and assistant will work 249 days minus 15 days or a total of 234 days per year. The number of anticipated units of productivity then for both departments is calculated as follows: 234 days × 10 therapists × 18 units or 42,120 units of treatment per year per department (see Table 4).

To simplify calculations both departments will be described as offering all services at the same price whether the service is evaluation or treatment. If the ten therapist department can generate 42,120 units of treatment per year and needs to produce $534,240 in revenue, the cost per unit of treatment would be $534,240 ÷ 42,120 units or $12.70/unit. In comparison, the five therapist, five assistant department must generate $443,712; therefore $443,712 ÷ 42,120 units equals $10.50 per unit. This yields a cost savings of $2.20/unit or $8.80/hour to the consumer, over the ten therapist department (see Table 5).

If these suggested costs per unit of treatment are much lower than the charges at your facility, remember that the mean annual incomes for therapists and assistants are based on a two-year-old survey and do not include the costs of fringe benefits. Also costs of the occupational therapy administrative staff, such as the occupational therapy director, senior occupational therapists, and secretaries who present *costs* to a department but little or no revenue were not included.

DISCUSSION

Before implementing new staffing patterns or recommending changes in existing configurations, the occupational therapy manager should first analyze the type of facility and the patient population within that facility targeted to receive occupational therapy services. If, for example, the services offered are primarily diagnostic in nature, the majority of staff will require expertise in administering evaluations and analyzing and interpreting the results. Thus, effective employment of assistants in this environment is minimal. If the occupational therapy department is located in an acute care hospital and physician referrals request evaluations, triage, and discharge planning, assistants may be of less value. Many other facilities, such as rehabilitation and home health agencies, nursing homes, and the public school system would clearly profit from the services of assistants. Funding for therapeutic services are often meager in these centers, making it difficult to hire qualified therapists. Consequently, such centers or facilities might hire a part-time therapist for evaluation and supervision purposes while employing full-time assistants for day to day treatment. This arrangement allows a center to provide quality patient care within the means of its available finances.

The occupational therapy manager must also consider primary sources for reimbursement. For instance, in some states, Medicaid will not reimburse for occupational therapy services provided by an assistant. This may be true of other 3rd party payors as well.

STRATEGIES FOR IMPLEMENTATION

Over the past year, the administrative staff at UTMB has considered these issues as the roles of several of our assistant positions have been redefined. Two staffing changes came about following analyses of both productivity standards and statistical results of occupational therapy services offered.

In the area of adult physical dysfunction, initial results concerning type of treatments rendered indicated that 54% of the treatments performed were under the service categories of activities of daily living or functional motor skills. The functional motor service category includes activities to improve range of motion, fine and gross motor coordination, and upper extremity strength. Twenty percent

Table 4

Total Annual Projected Departmental Productivity Based on Estimated Annual Chargeable Treatment Units.

Daily productivity X Number of therapists/assistants X
Number of annual working days = Estimated annual chargeable Treatment Units

18 Units (15 min. increments) X 10 therapists/assistants X
234 days (total working days minus 3 weeks combined vacation, administrative leave and sick days) = 42,120 Treatment Units

Table 5

A Comparison of Patient Charge Per 15 Minute Unit of Treatment Between an Occupational Therapy Department Comprised of All Therapists Versus a Department Comprised of Therapists and Assistants.

Department	Total Projected Costs ÷	Estimated Chargeable Units =	Patient Charge per Treatment Unit
One	$534,240	42,120 units	$12.70/unit
Two	443,712	42,120	10.50/unit
			$2.20/unit/$8.80 hr (savings to patient when treated by Department Two)

of evaluations were in daily living skills. These two categories of treatment and the one category of evaluation are appropriately performed by assistants. Yet, in general, the productivity of assistants at that time was less than that of therapists; thus, a question arose as to whether assistants were being used effectively or, if as was pointed out by both therapists and assistants, perhaps assistants were *assisting* with treatments and not generating their own units.

At the time of the initial analysis, four assistants were assigned to four of the six existing teams in adult physical dysfunction. One assistant in particular was treating patients through the outpatient clinic which primarily treats patients with hand injuries and cerebral vascular accidents. Numerous hand patients are seen through clinics and are seen one time only for evaluation and splinting or are rescheduled for extensive hand therapy. The other part of the patient load consists of patients who have suffered cerebral vascular accidents. These patients have often achieved independence in activities of daily living and are returning primarily for intensive muscle re-education of the upper limb. Busiest hours for the hand clinics requiring splinting is late morning and early afternoon.

The particular assistant assigned to the team, because of inability to treat the existing population, was unable to meet the defined productivity standards. She was reassigned to the geriatric rehabilitation program where the primary goal is the successful return of patients to home. Once evaluated, the assistant could perform self-care tasks training independently as well as reassess this particular patient population's progress.

The assistant just described is now responsible for patient care on the geriatric rehabilitation unit in the early morning and assists with patient care in the ambulatory care area during the busier clinic hours. Her day begins at 7:00 a.m. and ends at 4:00 p.m. Before initiating the above change in job routine, this assistant was averaging ten units of treatment daily. She presently averages eighteen units per day.

Analysis of occupational therapy services offered in the pediatric clinics at UTMB demonstrated that over 40% of the services consisted of evaluations of inpatients whose length of hospital stays were short. Upon discharge, patients often required referral to and coordination of services with other therapists in outside agencies. Staffing at this time consisted of five therapists and two assistants. Assistant productivity was twelve and eight units respectively.

The responsibilities of the assistant with the lowest productivity included the ordering and receiving of supplies, clinic maintenance, and fabrication of adaptive equipment for and treatment of chronically ill children. A decision was made to transfer this assistant to the acute care services in adult physical dysfunction where she would be responsible for an obstetrics group which consists of mothers who are at risk.

Treatment for the obstetrics patients is offered in a group atmosphere to offer emotional support and educational services regarding prenatal and postnatal care. The assistant is also responsible for group treatment to other patients having diagnoses which include diabetes, renal problems, and oncology. She offers support as well as activities to increase upper extremity strength, range of motion and coordination. She fabricates adaptive equipment and continues with some of her pediatric programming including the pediatric oncology support group. Her chargeable productivity now averages fifteen units daily as compared to eight units previously. Productivity for the assistant continuing full-time treatment in pediatrics has increased from twelve units to eighteen units daily.

CONCLUSION

In summary, assistants can be a valuable asset to many occupational therapy departments. Prior to implementing staffing changes, though, the occupational therapy manager should determine the benefit of such changes by utilizing cost accounting principles, reviewing the type of facility, the clientele to be served, occupational therapy services to be offered and the expertise of existing staff.

REFERENCES

American Occupational Therapy Association (1986). *Manpower commission report*. Rockville, MD: Author.

American Occupational Therapy Association (1987). 1986 member data survey (Interim report #1). Rockville, MD: Author.

American Occupational Therapy Association (1987). COTAs today. *Occupational Therapy News, 41*(6), 11-14.

Brooks, B. (1982). COTA issues: Yesterday, today and tomorrow. *American Journal of Occupational Therapy, 36*(9), 567-568.

Strickland, L. R. (1988). Career ladder development for certified occupational therapy assistants. *Occupational Therapy in Health Care, 5*(2/3), 7-21.

Designing Job Enrichment Projects

Gail Lacey Clakeley, OTR

SUMMARY. This paper describes a management strategy for a job satisfaction program utilized in a large occupational therapy department. The goal of the program is to retain satisfied, productive employees and reduce attrition of therapists and assistants. The use of job enrichment projects for occupational therapy assistants will be presented with brief descriptions of two projects.

INTRODUCTION

Job satisfaction is a significant factor influencing an individual's decision to remain in a given work situation. Occupational therapy managers have the capacity to take an active role in facilitating and designing job enrichment activities for therapists and assistants. Several factors can be considered when job enrichment is utilized: length of time in a given job, the amount of challenge and opportunity the work provides, compatibility between employee interests and programmatic concerns, and the capacity for management to provide a vertical mobility system that financially recognizes performance. This paper describes a plan used to enhance job enrichment for certified occupational therapy assistants at the University of Texas Medical Branch (UTMB) Hospital in Galveston, Texas.

Gail Lacey Clakeley has a baccalaureate degree from Northeast Louisiana University. She is currently Assistant Director for Psychiatry/Pediatrics in the Department of Occupational Therapy at the University of Texas Medical Branch in Galveston, TX.

The support and encouragement of Lillian Hoyle Parent, OTR and L. Randy Strickland, OTR is gratefully acknowledged.

This article appears jointly in *Certified Occupational Therapy Assistants: Opportunities and Challenges* (The Haworth Press, 1988) and *Occupational Therapy in Health Care*, Volume 5, Numbers 2/3 (1988).

JOB SATISFACTION

Although many factors influence a person's decision to remain on a job, such as pay and pleasant work environments, job satisfaction is the most prominent factor. Cada (1981) states that identification of intrinsic motivators should indicate specific action steps to plan and evaluate the climate for job enrichment. Two of Cada's hypotheses can be utilized as a sound basis for planning job enrichment programs for certified occupational therapy assistants (hereinafter referred to as assistants) and are described below.

1. Job satisfaction is positively related to an individual's decision to remain in a given setting. For example, at the University of Texas Medical Branch the total length of employment for ten assistants currently on staff is 57 years; this was the first job for 6 of the 10 assistants. Attrition over the last 4 years has been approximately 15%.
2. Differences in job satisfaction are found between therapists who have worked less than two years and those who have worked longer. Specifically, identified differences relate to skill variety, task significance, feedback from the job, internal work motivation, pay, security, and social supervisor and growth satisfaction.

Cada, citing Maslow (1954), reported that only needs not yet satisfied can influence behavior and therefore can be considered motivators. An adequately fulfilled need is not a motivator, and once a particular need is fulfilled another emerges and demands fulfillment. This is illustrated by socialization, which is an important motivator for a new employee but is less of a motivator for a more experienced employee. For example, managers who feel they are constantly "feeding" their staff should understand that this is a normal developmental pattern and does not suggest that they or their employees are inadequate. Another example is found in the expansion of clinical specializations in occupational therapy. Regardless of a department's philosophy or policy regarding specialization, "status" is associated with therapists who specialize.

One strategy to maintain or increase job satisfaction is the utilization of individually designed job enrichment projects. These projects can be discussed and designed as part of the routine employee evaluation procedure. The natural collaborative relationship between assistants and registered occupational therapists (hereinafter referred to as therapists) is ideal for planning job enrichment projects that mutually benefit assistants, therapists, and patients.

JOB ENRICHMENT

Psychologist Ernest Becker, (cited in Peters & Waterman, 1982) states that "man is driven by his essential 'dualism,' he needs *both* to be a part something and to 'stick out,' " (p. xxi). Humans at one and the same time need to be conforming members of a winning team and to be stars in their own right. To fulfill individuals' needs to make unique contributions, the UTMB occupational therapy department incorporates the development of individual special projects/goals into an annual review process which gives the manager input from the assistant in identifying intrinsic motivators.

In addition to regularly assigned duties, each staff member at our facility is required to select or design a special project. This project reflects interests of individual staff members and meets programmatic needs or concerns (Puccetti, 1988). The manager can guide the employee with skills and aptitudes but no identified special interest by identifying special projects that fulfill program needs and goals. Assistants have an opportunity to view their jobs as having a broader scope and as contributing to the departments overall plan, and the manager makes a commitment to allow assistants to initiate and complete their projects.

To insure the success of job enrichment projects several characteristics can be considered: longevity and retention, challenge, opportunity, experience or vertical mobility and compatibility. Each characteristic will be discussed.

Longevity and Retention

Assistants in the occupational therapy department at the UTMB are far less mobile than are therapists. As assistants increase their longevity in the same jobs they have a higher risk of becoming less productive as their workload becomes more routine. Rather than accept the "fate" of long term employees, the job enrichment program promotes the concept of some degree of autonomy in practice and fosters development of greater clinical depth and competency. This is done without overloading the assistants or requesting them to do work that requires the skills of a therapist.

Challenge

There is a fine line between staff development and staff overload. When employees design their own programs and set their own schedules of completion, they experience a sense of control over their work. This prevents frustration and decreased motivation resulting from a subjective experience of having little or no control over one's job or work environment. Allowing employees to design and schedule part of their jobs requires greater flexibility and more far-sighted planning on the part of the manager.

Opportunity

Many times assistants have more time available than do therapists for in-depth development of treatment techniques. Rapid patient turnover in an acute service often requires therapists to devote considerable time to evaluation and documentation. Therapists are also involved in more meetings, rounds, and student training programs. This creates opportunities for the assistant to plan treatment regimens that can be developed, approved and carried out independently or with minimal supervision.

Experience or Vertical Mobility

Many therapists are promoted to senior status after 2-3 years of clinical experience. Vertical mobility is not always an option for assistants so implementation of a promotion system that can financially recognize senior status for assistants helps immensely in recognizing their contributions. UTMB has been able to incorporate a system that allows for an entry level position of COTA I and a senior position of COTA II. The special project is utilized as an opportunity for assistants to develop advanced skills and the broader scope of knowledge required in the senior assistant position.

Compatibility

Compatibility is the matching of jobs with an individual's interests or skills. There are infinite parameters for this and unlimited opportunities for creativity in this area. Patient and program needs can be matched with individual interests and skills. For example, a substance abuse program needing a 7:00 a.m. exercise class can be matched with an assistant who wishes to attend evening classes to pursue a bachelor's degree.

Consideration of the above factors can facilitate the manager's capacity to individualize job enrichment projects. The projects can be selected based on the needs of individual assistants at a given time. Managers can respond to changes in professional development and the personal situations of each employee. The assistants' need to provide a unique contribution and receive recognition for their work experience can be met through individually designed job enrichment projects.

EXAMPLES OF JOB ENRICHMENT PROJECTS

When assistants are given the opportunity to develop their own projects, based on identified needs (their own as well as those of patients and the program), their overall investment to the specific program is greater. This level of personal satisfaction seems to influence other aspects of their work. For example, as assistants in our facility have been perceived as being capable of developing and implementing activities, versus implementing activities developed by others, they have volunteered for responsibilities (i.e., participation in career days, health fairs, professional orientations, or student seminars) that require greater leadership skills. Consequently, therapists and higher levels of administration have become more knowledgeable regarding the skills of assistants and are more likely to select or request them for specific tasks.

One assistant developed a job readiness program that includes training in the basic skills required to obtain or maintain a job (Wassink, 1988). Following a therapist's assessment and recommendation that a patient requires greater skill in the area of work preparation, the patient is referred to this assistant. The assistant uses discretion within the parameters of the approved protocol (all treatment protocols pass a multi-therapist review process) to carry out or conduct the job readiness program. To illustrate, another assistant often serves as consultant to several programs and therapists in adapting a variety of toys for patients. This assistant developed the skill of toy adaptation in response to two separate events. The pediatric rehabilitation unit had suffered a serious decrease in patient census creating a problem with staff productivity. At the same time a recreational therapist in the program found information about toy adaptation and asked the assistant if she might be interested in learning the techniques. She became more involved and excited about the project and was able to identify specific patients who could benefit from having toys adapted (Lemire, 1988).

Within the realm of treatment protocols, both of these assistants just described have developed areas of expertise for which they have received recognition and "status" associated with technical or specialty competence. Both individuals have also been recognized by professionals outside of the Occupational Therapy Department. The first assistant was invited to give a lecture and conduct a laboratory session in a baccalaureate degree program, and she presented a paper at a state conference. The Occupational Therapy Department has also received letters of commendation regarding her performance with patients from representatives of referring agencies. The second assistant described above was an exhibitor for toy adaptations at a recent Texas Medical Association Conference.

CONCLUSION

Job enrichment projects are a management strategy to promote job satisfaction. The utilization of job enrichment projects fosters individual growth and initiative, and promotes accomplishment of clinical competence. This management strategy allows flexibility in staffing, anticipates needs for creative programming, and most importantly, fosters and retains productive, satisfied certified occupational therapy assistants.

REFERENCES

Cada, E.A. (1981). *Occupational therapy: A diagnostic survey*. Unpublished master's thesis. George Williams College. Downers Grove, IL.

Lemire, E. (1988). Toy adaptations in pediatrics. *Occupational Therapy in Health Care, 5*(2/3), 87-97.

Maslow, A. (1954). *Motivation and personality*. New York: Harper and Row.

Peters, T.J., Waterman, R.H., Jr. (1982). *In search of excellence*. New York: Warner Books.

Puccetti, D.D. (1988). Supervision of the COTA: Developing a knowledge base. *Occupational Therapy in Health Care, 5*(2/3), 23-35.

Wassink, K.E. (1988). Job search skills for unemployed psychiatric patients. *Occupational Therapy in Health Care, 5*(2/3), 149-158.

Certified Occupational Therapy Assistants and Microcomputers

Barbara J. Brewer, COTA
Penni McMahon, COTA

SUMMARY. This article deals with the continually changing role of the Certified Occupational Therapy Assistant. When the need for Registered Occupational Therapists became greater than the number of available therapists, a program was instituted for assistants. At first these aides, as they were called at that time, were delegated the tasks of transporting patients to and from therapy and setting them up for therapy. Gradually, the assistant's role grew, and with the emergence of the team approach, the assistant's role changed once again. Today the assistant is a valuable member of the team and by specializing can enhance the quality of care provided for the patient.

One area of specialization is computer-assisted therapy. The assistant can enhance the quality of care provided and offer a different treatment approach. This article will review software in current use at Rancho Los Amigos Medical Center and the involvement of assistants in computer-assisted therapy.

INTRODUCTION

For the past three years the Occupational Therapy assistants at Rancho Los Amigos Medical Center have been involved in computer-assisted therapy for perceptual and cognitive retraining. In the

---

Barbara J. Brewer is a staff COTA at Rancho Los Amigos Medical Center, Downey, CA, on the Neuro/Stroke Service. Penni McMahon is a staff COTA at Rancho Los Amigos Medical Center on the Spinal Cord Injury Service. Questions regarding information from this article may be sent to: Barbara J. Brewer, COTA, c/o 800 Occupational Therapy, Rm. 36, Rancho Los Amigos Medical Center, 7601 East Imperial Highway, Downey, CA 90242.

This article appears jointly in *Certified Occupational Therapy Assistants: Opportunities and Challenges* (The Haworth Press, 1988) and *Occupational Therapy in Health Care*, Volume 5, Numbers 2/3 (1988).

past microcomputers have been utilized in therapy as games or as diversional therapy. More recently, however, increasing numbers of software programs have been written to assist with treatment or rehabilitation programs. These software programs can assist the therapy team with evaluation, treatment, pre-vocational testing and training and can be incorporated into traditional treatment modalities to enhance the effectiveness of care provided by occupational therapists.

ROLE OF THE COTA

In 1949 the increasing need for registered occupational therapists led to development of programs for certified occupational therapy assistants. At first these aides, as they were called, worked in the psychiatric setting. They provided the patients with activities under the supervision of therapists who served as consultants. In the early 1960s needs for assistant programs in nursing homes became apparent, and thus a program was begun to prepare assistants for work with these patients. Prior to 1965, the assistant working in physical dysfunction was assigned such tasks as transporting and preparing patients for treatment. The assistant was not expected to, and did not make, decisions independently of therapists. In the 1970s the role of assistants changed considerably. They assumed visible roles in AOTA as well as on the job. Assistants were given more responsibility and were asked to become more involved in the overall treatment of patients. With the emergence of the team approach assistants found themselves thrust into the treatment program as partners with therapists and again were asked to make more changes in their approach. Assistants today have to be more assertive in their interaction with therapists. They must demonstrate to therapists that they are capable of assisting therapists in determining the treatment program best suited for patients. The experienced assistant can, and does, make decisions related to treatment planning and implementation on an ongoing basis.

As with therapists, assistants can also specialize in different treatment modalities. One type of specialization is in the area of computer-assisted therapy. By becoming familiar with the use of microcomputers the assistant can enhance the quality of care provided and offer a different treatment approach for the patient. In order for the assistant to effectively carry out a treatment program utilizing the computer some prerequisites should be met. The assistant should have at least one year of experience in acute rehabilitation and/or a basic understanding of the philosophy of the rehabilitation process. He or she should have a working knowledge of the microcomputer and be able to explain its use to other staff and patients.

At Rancho Los Amigos Medical Center, the therapy team sets objectives and goals for the patient and at that time determines if the computer can be incorporated into the treatment program to accomplish these goals. The assistant then has the task of selecting the appropriate programs and carrying out the treatment program that addresses these specific goals.

MICROCOMPUTERS IN THERAPY

The assistant can use the computer as a substitute for some traditional evaluation tools, such as paper and pencil tests, if they are suitable to the patient's specific needs or deficits. Programs such as the *Visual/Perceptual Diagnostic Testing and Training Program*[6] from Educational Electronic Techniques, Ltd., is an example of this. This program allows the team greater latitude in the evaluation procedure. The computer can also be used to work on cognitive skills such as increasing attention span, memory, and problem solving.

The specific computer program selected is not meant to be a replacement for conventional therapy but rather as an assist to enhance the therapy program. An added feature that makes use of a microcomputer valuable is that it is objective rather than subjective. The computer does not make judgements as to how the task was completed but rather is concerned with task completion. Many programs may have a built-in printer option; results can be printed out and included in the patient's chart and/or stored on a disk for future reference. Since the data is objective rather than subjective, it is, therefore, more consistent in its interpretation. Thus the assistant has objective data to write in her running notes, which provides validity for the content of her notes.

Although computer software is usually appropriate for most patients, adaptations are needed for some to allow them to participate in computer-assisted therapy. The assistant works with the therapist and the patient in choosing, designing or fabricating equipment that allows the patient to use peripherals which were previously inaccessible.

The assistant can also incorporate the computer into a behavior modification program. It can be used as a reward after a patient has completed a difficult task or toward the end of a therapy session. An example of this is allowing a patient with a head trauma to use *Print Shop*[3] by Broderbund, to make a sign or *County Fair*[8] by Data Most for enjoyment. This allows the patient to have some control over his program with consequences for failure to comply with its instructions.

EVALUATION

The microcomputer can assist the therapy team with evaluations of a variety of visual/perceptual problems: visual tracking, visual scanning, spatial relations and figure ground. It can also be used as an assistive tool to evaluate neglect, motor planning problems, and cognitive skills such as attention span, memory and problem solving.

Often patients are unable to complete paper/pencil tests that are secondary to motor planning problems and/or other deficits that interfere with function. In these instances software designed by Educational Electronics Techniques, Ltd., is used. The series of disks titled *Visual/Perceptual Diagnostic Testing and Training Program*[6] allows the assistant to assess the patient's ability in the areas of visual discrimination, visual memory, figure ground, spatial relations and scanning. The assistant selects the appropriate response mode for this program, which is designed for use with the Gibson Light Pen, the space bar, or a micro-switch to allow the patient an opportunity to complete the task with ease. The therapist can interpret the data from the print-out and together with the assistant determine what areas needs to be addressed during treatment. In this way the computer is used to assist with the treatment program.

At Rancho Los Amigos Medical Center the assistant often chooses the programs that are best suited to the patients' needs.

Other software that can be used for evaluation includes *Cognitive Education Series*[10] by Karl Lambert and *Psychological Software Service*[2] programs for cognitive rehabilitation by Odie Bracy, PhD. These programs vary in their approach to evaluation but provide a variety of therapeutic evaluation tools for the therapy team.

For the stroke patient the programs from Educational Electronics Techniques, Ltd., are best suited for use as an evaluation tool. The programs from *Cognitive Education Series*[10] and *Psychological Software Services*[2] are geared more towards patients with cognitive deficits such as those associated with head trauma or spinal cord injury with a secondary diagnosis of closed head trauma.

TREATMENT

A multitude of programs exist that can be used for treatment. We will address some of those programs that the assistants at Rancho Los Amigos Medical Center have found to be most effective for use with our patients. Although three distinct and different diagnoses are addressed in this article, most of these programs can be used to enhance therapy programs for the following problems regardless of diagnosis: visual/perceptual problems, decreased problem solving, decreased memory, and scanning deficits.

Conventional therapy for neglect and/or visual field deficits positions the task in the area where the deficit occurs. The patient then attends to the task by looking to the side on which the deficit exists to complete the task. When using the computer the patient is positioned in front of the monitor in midline position. By loading a program designed to give responses in all four visual quadrants, the patient is encouraged to scan the screen to complete the required task. The advantage of this program is that a response mode is built into it that provides objective data about how well the patient responded to the stimuli in all four visual quadrants. It provides a print-out, if needed, for the Occupational Therapy chart. These programs are also applicable for use as scanning tasks: "Visual Scanning II" by Educational Electronics Techniques, Ltd., *Foundation Skills*[2] by Psychological Software Services and a program called *Connection*[1] which resembles the board game entitled *Connect 4.*[12]

The computer gives patients an opportunity to become actively involved in problem solving and decision making. Examples of problem solving and decision making activities that are carried out during traditional therapy are having a head trauma patient plan a meal, a stroke patient open a container with one hand or a spinal cord injury patient select adaptive equipment. With the computer the assistant can also choose from a variety of programs that address problem solving and decision making tasks, including involvement of the patient in selecting the appropriate program. Programs that can be related to the above activities are found on *Managing Lifestyles: Survival Math Skills*[14] by Sunburst Communications. This program is designed to work on computation skills and is modeled on real-life situations for budgeting for groceries, budgeting living expenses and meal preparation.

As the computer is not designed for opening containers a different type of program may be chosen. An example of a simple problem solving program is called "Layer Cake" on the *Mix and Match*[4] from CTW disk in which a cake with three layers is moved from one plate to another without putting a larger layer on top of a smaller layer. Similarly the assistant may also choose a program from *Cognitive Education Series*[10] disk number two, entitled "Stack Up." This program is more difficult as it requires the patient to move a stack of four layers from table one to table three without putting a larger layer on top of a smaller layer. The program offers the patient the opportunity to escape if the task becomes too frustrating. As with "Layer Cake" the number of moves required to transfer the stack is displayed. This number can be recorded in the Occupational Therapy chart for future reference. Some other types of programs used for problem solving include *Trolls Tale*[16] by Sierra On-Line, *The Factory*[9] from Sunburst Communications, *Oregon Trail*[13] by Minnesota Educational Computing Consortium and *Cognitive Education Series*[10] by Lambert. Spinal cord injury patients can also benefit from these problem solving programs as many have a secondary diagnosis of head trauma. Assistants use the objective data from these programs in their written reports to the supervising therapists.

In the hospital setting, neurologically involved patients have little or no choice as to when they get up, what they eat, or when they go to therapy. Even their bowel and bladder care is on a schedule.

Programs such as *Print Shop*[3] enable patients with spinal cord injuries the opportunity to make their own decisions. This program provides choices as to what they make (i.e., a sign, greeting card or banner) and its content. In this way, the assistant can evaluate some simple problem solving and decision making skills as well. Since motivation and depression are common problems with the spinal cord injury patient this form of therapeutic activity can be helpful in enabling the patient to feel better about himself.

There are a variety of memory programs that can be used with most patients. Examples of these programs are "Master Match" by Cognitive Education Series, "Visual Memory" from Educational Electronics Techniques, Ltd., *Memory I and II*[2] by Psychological Software Service, and *Memory Castle*[18] from Sunburst Communications. Most programs are designed to be graded from simple to more complex levels with each level requiring the patient to remember increasing numbers of items.

PRE-VOCATIONAL TRAINING

Typing training is one of the typical treatment areas for patients with spinal cord injuries. It works well because it is a familiar task, and most patients realize the job potential one has with good typing skills. Typing is also an activity that can lead to a vocation with computers and word processing.

Patients with all levels of spinal cord injuries can learn typing. For example, the patient with no neck mobility can type using a tongue activated protractable mouth stick; a patient with an injury at the C-4 level can use a straight or static mouth stick. Patients with C-5 level injuries can use a ratchet orthosis or a writing device with a wrist support, with or without mobile arm supports. With a C-6 level injury, a patient uses universal cuffs, a wrist driven wrist hand orthosis, or different types of writing or typing devices. The assistant spends considerable time with the patient trying to find and select adaptive equipment that works best for each patient and to train her. This is a good opportunity for the patient to become familiar with different types of equipment that may be used in other activities such as writing, feeding, and hygiene and grooming.

Use of computers offers the patient an avenue of expression that may have been difficult or inaccessible previously. As with any new learning experience the assistant may find he has to spend considerable time with the patient teaching them to use the computer. *Master Type*[19] by Scarborough Systems, Inc., is a good typing program for patients who have fine motor control for it enables patients to practice and improve their typing skills. This is especially appropriate for the patient who prior to his injury did much typing. A word processing program called *Appleworks*[11] by Apple Computer, Inc., is more effective for the beginning typist. With this program it is not necessary for the patient to look at the monitor when typing. Instead, the patient can concentrate on hitting the keys and when finished can review, correct typing mistakes, and print the document. The assistant needs to intervene when patients tend to look from the keyboard to the monitor to check for spelling errors and suggest ways to make the activity less frustrating.

There are a number of keyboard adaptions commercially available for *Appleworks*[11] that make it possible for patients with all levels of spinal cord injuries to use with special keyboard adaptations that are now readily available. The patient with decreased hand function or with only one functional extremity can effectively use the computer for vocational tasks. Computer-assisted therapy for the patient with a stroke or head trauma serves as pre-vocational skills training in that it allows the patient to work on problem solving and decision making skills.

DISCUSSION

The assistant today must be assertive and develop competency to compete successfully in the occupational therapy profession. With advanced competency the assistant gains increased job satisfaction and personal self-esteem which carries over into areas of job performance. Computer-assisted therapy is a specialization with which the assistant can become a valuable member of the team. By developing competency in computer-assisted therapy many become instructors and resource persons for the occupational therapy department, thereby gaining the respect of the other therapy staff and contributing to an improvement in the quality of therapy offered by the department.

CONCLUSION

The assistants at Rancho Los Amigos Medical Center are becoming more involved in computer-assisted therapy and are responsible for incorporating the computer in therapy. Assistants spend considerable time with patients selecting programs that would be most beneficial for the patient to achieve their goals.

Thus, by developing expertise the assistant can be an effective and valuable member of the therapy team. As a group, assistants need to expand their roles and responsibilities.

NOTES

1. Anderson, C. (1979). *Connection* (Computer program). Raleigh, NC.
2. Bracy, O. *Psychological Software Service Programs for Cognitive Rehabilitation* (Computer program). Indianapolis, IN: Psychological Software Service.
3. Broderbund Software, Inc. (1984). *Print Shop* (Computer program). San Rafael, CA: Broderbund Software, Inc.
4. CTW. *Mix and Match*. (Computer program). Cupertino, CA: Apple Computer, Inc.
5. Garcia, Greenfield (1981). Dynamic Protractable Mouth, *American Journal of Occupational Therapy, 35*, 8.
6. Greenbush, Chamoff (1985). *Visual-Perceptual Diagnostic Testing and Training Program* (Computer program). Wantagh, NY: Educational Electronics Techniques, Limited.
7. Hirama, H. (1986). The COTA A Chronological Review. In S. Ryan (Ed.), *The Certified Occupational Therapy Assistant Roles and Responsibilities*. (pg. 22-34) NJ: Slack Inc.
8. Illowski, D. (1981). *County Fair* (Computer program). Data Most.
9. Kosel, M. and Fish, M. (1986). *The Factory* (Computer program). Pleasantville, NY: Sunburst Communications.
10. Lambert, K. (1983). *Cognitive Educational System* (Computer program). Chula Vista, CA: Cognitive Educational Series.
11. Lissner, R. (1983). *Appleworks* (Computer program). Cupertino, CA: Apple Computer, Inc., VI, 1, USA.
12. Milton Bradley. *Connect 4* (Board game). Springfield, MA: Milton Bradley.

13. Minnesota Educational Computing Consortium. *Oregon Trail*. St. Paul, MN: Minnesota Educational Computing Consortium.

14. Near, M. (1986). *Managing Lifestyles: Survival Math Skills*. Pleasantville, NY: Sunburst Communications.

15. Sidler, M. (1986). Computer applications in occupational therapy. *Occupational Therapy in Health Care, 3*, 3-4.

16. Sierra On-Line (1984). *Trolls Tale*. Coarsegold, CA: Sierra On-Line, Inc.

17. Siev, E., Freishtat, B., & Zoltan, B. (1986). *Perceptual and Cognitive Dysfunction in the Adult Stroke Patient*. Slack, Inc.

18. Stanger, D. (1984). *Memory Castle* (Computer program) Pleasantville, NY: Sunburst Communications Rochester School District, Rochester, MN.

19. Zweig, B. (1983). *Master Type* (Computer program). Scarborough Systems, Inc.

SOFTWARE SOURCES

CONNECTION (sometimes called Connect Four). Original program by Chip Anderson (9/12/79), 404 Vernon Terrace, Raleigh, NC 27609. Phone (919) 781-4229. Connection is also included in Classic Apple Disk #1, available for $10 from Computer Using Educators (CUE) Softswap, P.O. Box 271704, Concord, CA 94527-1704.

LAYER CAKE is included on the "Mix and Match" disk which includes Layer Cake, Animals, Raise the Flag, and Sesame Street Muppets Mix and Max. Copyright 1981 by CTW. Requires 64K Apple and is better with a color monitor. For information contact Alan Brightman, Special Education Office, Apple Computer Inc., 20525 Mariani Avenue, Cupertino, CA 95041. Phone (408) 996-1010.

STACK-UP, a more advanced version of Layer Cake, is available from Karl Lambert, Cognitive Educational Series. Requires 64K Apple and monochrome monitor. Mr. Lambert has recently moved. Call Ramona, CA (619) 789-1438.

THE OREGON TRAIL is produced by Minnesota Educational Computing Corporation (MECC), 3490 Lexington Avenue North, St. Paul, MN 55126. Phone (612) 481-3500. Requires 64K Apple. Color monitor preferable. No. A-157. $49.

GENERAL RESOURCES IN SPECIAL EDUCATION

Closing the Gap, P.O. Box 68, Henderson, MN 56044. Phone (612) 248-3294. One year newsletter subscription is $21.

Special Education Software Center. For software information call 1(800)327-5893. Sponsored by the U.S. Department of Education, Special Education Programs.

Wheelchair Clinics Work

Jo-Ann Brant

SUMMARY. The positioning problems and needs of severely disabled adults greatly influence their ability to function independently. This paper will describe an interdisciplinary approach in a wheelchair clinic, the functions of a wheelchair clinic, and the role of a Certified Occupational Therapy Assistant as part of the wheelchair clinic team.

Approximately two and a half years ago, the staff of the Adult Day Treatment Program at United Cerebral Palsy Association of Western New York, Inc., noted that increasing numbers of clients were poorly positioned in their wheelchairs or needed equipment that would ensure functional positions for daily activities. It was also known that the process of ordering and justifying proper durable medical equipment required time-consuming efforts, especially on the part of the occupational therapist.

In reviewing and estimating wheelchair needs among the agency's clients, it was concluded that space was available in the facility for a wheelchair clinic and that the facility could effectively service wheelchair clients. Consequently, a decision was made to develop a wheelchair clinic, which was instituted in 1985. It has now evolved

---

Jo-Ann Brant holds an Associate Degree in Applied Science and is a certified occupational therapy assistant at the United Cerebral Palsy Association of Western New York, Inc. Additional information can be obtained from Ms. Brant by writing her at the United Cerebral Palsy Association of Western New York, Inc., 7 Community Drive, Buffalo, NY 14225.

The continuing support and inspiration of Jan Nowak, OTR/L, which enabled me to work in the Wheelchair Clinic is gratefully acknowledged.

This article appears jointly in *Certified Occupational Therapy Assistants: Opportunities and Challenges* (The Haworth Press, 1988) and *Occupational Therapy in Health Care*, Volume 5, Numbers 2/3 (1988).

to service not only day treatment clients but also clients referred from other agencies and resources in the community.

This presentation will discuss the purposes and functions of the Wheelchair Clinic, the responsibilities of the Certified Occupational Therapy Assistant (COTA) in the Wheelchair Clinic, and the contributions of the interdisciplinary team which support the Wheelchair Clinic.

THE WHEELCHAIR CLINIC

The Wheelchair Clinic provides clients with the opportunity to experiment with the most up-to-date durable medical equipment before purchase decisions are made. During this period of exploration input is sought from the client and from members of the interdisciplinary team, such as physicians, therapists, teachers, family members, and other related professionals. Information from all of these sources ensures that a wheelchair is selected which best suits the needs of the individual and provides sufficient professional guidance for the client to be positioned functionally in the new wheelchair. After decisions are made about the most appropriate equipment for the client's needs, staff in the Wheelchair Clinic adjust the wheelchair so that it properly fits the client.

The Wheelchair Clinic has numerous resources available for trial use by the clients, including a variety of cushions, custom inserts, foot supports, and custom chest straps and seat belts. Cushions may be used by a client for one week trial periods so that the client knows whether or not any given cushion will meet his physical needs, such as protecting pressure points, facilitating the client's ability to transfer, or providing functional support to the ischial tuberosities and coccyx.

Custom inserts, such as lateral, head and neck supports are available for special clients with many physical needs, as are foot supports. Foot supports maintain the lower extremities functionally in a 90 degree angle or other appropriate position and include toe, heel, and ankle straps with foot rests which have adjustable angles to provide adequate support for the feet.

Custom chest straps and seat belts are made within the wheelchair clinic to fit the patient functionally in the midline. Custom lap trays can be purchased to enhance the client's ability to carry out daily living skills, such as feeding himself, handling speech devices, and conducting other therapeutic activities.

Having a variety of equipment and supplies available for trial use in the wheelchair clinic, as well as the availability of trained personnel to make custom items or to adapt items to meet a client's particular needs, provides a valuable service to clients and their families.

THE COTA's ROLE IN THE WHEELCHAIR CLINIC

The COTA performs many important and supportive roles in the operation of the Wheelchair Clinic, including preparation and writing of medical justifications for the equipment, communicating with attending and Wheelchair Clinic physicians, and scheduling appointments for the Clinic and for wheelchair repairs.

Third party payment is usually required for purchase of durable medical equipment. The COTA writes the medical justifications, and because of the abundance of justifications required for each clinic, the assistant is familiar with the terminology required to obtain the particular type of durable medical equipment required for any given patient.

The COTA notifies the attending physician and the wheelchair physician when writing the medical justifications and discusses the recommendations of the Wheelchair Clinic team for specific types of equipment with the physicians. The physician(s) then signs the required forms and justifications.

All appointments and referrals from other agencies are handled by the COTA. This enables the Wheelchair Clinic to run smoothly within the amount of time allotted for proper evaluation by the Wheelchair Clinic interdisciplinary team. The COTA also schedules wheelchair repairs for the repairman. There have been increasing needs for wheelchair repairs, most of which are done in the Clinic in one day, thereby providing better servicing for the client.

Finally, the COTA works with medical vendors, who are an important part of the Wheelchair Clinic and who provide information to the Wheelchair Clinic teams about the availability of updated medical equipment. This helps the team make proper recommendations for the client.

The COTA's role in the Wheelchair Clinic is one of coordinating the necessary and vital support activities that enable the Clinic to run smoothly and effectively and to meet the particular needs of its clients.

THE INTERDISCIPLINARY TEAM

Before ordering or purchasing a wheelchair, an interdisciplinary team, consisting of therapists, assistants, physicians, teachers, aides, parents, and/or medical vendors, ensures that the wheelchair will functionally fit a client's needs. Considerations must include proper body alignment, placements of the head, trunk, legs, feet, and arms, and weight distribution. Many clients with handicaps need assistance in changing positions, and when placed in their best and most functional positions, they must be comfortable and be able to function independently.

CONCLUSION

Since the Wheelchair Clinic was established in March, 1985, 200 adults with disabilities have been serviced. Of these 200 clients serviced, 125 received new wheelchairs, 85 received adaptive equipment, and 75 received repairs and adaptations to existing wheelchairs. The success of the Wheelchair Clinic has given the author opportunity to lecture about positioning of adults with disabilities at state conferences, medical facility staff in-service meetings, and at area colleges.

Splinting Design and Fabrication in Physical Disabilities: A Splinting Assistance Program

Imelda Padilla, COTA

SUMMARY. An experienced Certified Occupational Therapy Assistant describes an identified need for splinting education for occupational therapists and students working in a multiclinic department. The occupational therapists, who are all responsible for treating patients on weekends and holidays, needed to maintain competency and consistency in completing splinting requests for a wide variety of medical and surgical services in a teaching hospital. The methods for developing and implementing a quarterly inservice program and its results are described.

INTRODUCTION

This paper will describe a special project which has been implemented because of the experience and interest of a Certified Occupational Therapy Assistant (COTA) in hand splinting. The assistant has ten years of experience in psychiatry and physical disabilities. For the last five years, the COTA has been on a treatment team assigned to patients referred from the burn, orthopedic surgery and plastic surgery services.

Imelda Padilla is assigned to the Texas Department of Correction Hospital and the Plastic and Orthopedic Surgery and Burn Services in the Department of Occupational Therapy at the University of Texas Medical Branch Hospitals. She is a graduate of Galveston Community College.

This article appears jointly in *Certified Occupational Therapy Assistants: Opportunities and Challenges* (The Haworth Press, 1988) and *Occupational Therapy in Health Care,* Volume 5, Numbers 2/3 (1988).

BACKGROUND

Several factors led to development of this hand splinting program. Each will be discussed briefly. Assistance in splinting was often sought from team members less experienced in splinting or by therapists on other teams because the treatment team had much experience in preparing splints. Although the burn, orthopedics and plastic surgery team members were willing to provide the assistance, this did not encourage development of independence in splinting skills among other therapists.

Because of the size of this particular teaching hospital there are numerous service areas, each with its own set of physicians and residents. Each physician and service area often has its own idiosyncracies and preferred methods of splinting. The splinting assistance program was designed to collect and share information from these various services with all staff. Finally, with the implementation of Saturday and holiday coverage, it was decided that all staff should be familiar with special needs and requests of specific physicians. Furthermore, a decision was made to have all staff acquire experience in fabrication of some of the splints that might be requested.

PROGRAM DEVELOPMENT

From analysis of these needs and problems, the Splinting Assistance Program was developed and now is offered quarterly. The main objective of this program was to increase therapists' knowledge of physicians' preferences and nomenclature so that fewer calls would be necessary by therapists to physicians when consultations arrived. Improvement in splinting skills, and knowledge of a given physician's preferences would decrease the number of revisions required following fabrication of splints.

The specific goals of the program were to:

1. increase O.T. staff and student knowledge and skills of splinting techniques through lecture and experiential learning;
2. increase use of uniform terminology when referring to splints and materials within the department; and

3. educate staff about particular splinting requests which might be received from the various physicians and service areas referring patients to occupational therapy.

The content of each workshop is based on information received from a questionnaire submitted to staff members. The questionnaire obtains information from staff regarding splints they view as being problematic. Specific questions allow staff to address specific topics about splinting materials, techniques and/or specific difficulties they have experienced when attempting particular splint fabrication. Therapists are also encouraged to list available days and times for attending a workshop that will address these specific issues.

Once questionnaires are returned the assistant tabulates the data to determine which splints will be most appropriate for presentations. Handouts are compiled for each splint to be demonstrated in the workshop, and patterns and directions for fabrication of the splints are included in the handouts (Cannon, Foltz, Koepfer, Lauck, Simpson, Bromley, 1985; Malick, 1975). Other information includes points about correct fit of the splint, its placement and wearing times.

The workshops are conducted quarterly for two hours each session. The first half hour of the workshop is a lecture by the assistant followed by a question and answer session. The other hour and a half allows for hands-on practical application of information reviewed in the lecture on splinting techniques and materials. Prior to the workshop all participants are asked to bring supplies and tools from their assigned work areas for the portion of the workshop devoted to splint fabrication. Participants are asked to use scrap thermoplastic splint materials for these exercises to conserve expensive supplies.

After the lecture, participants are placed in small groups, each headed by an experienced therapist or assistant, and are allowed time to fabricate each splint selected for that workshop. This portion of the workshop allows the new or inexperienced therapist an opportunity to practice using the information just received in a nonthreatening situation away from patients and physicians.

OUTCOMES

The organization of the workshops has proven to be successful in that participants have the opportunity to apply the information just received, to work with a variety of materials, and to receive immediate feedback and suggestions to facilitate fabrication of each splint covered in the particular workshop.

The Splinting Assistance Program has been evaluated through verbal feedback from the participants and an evaluation form is currently being developed. In the last year and a half the assistant has been requested to repeat this program six times, and the number of staff participants has increased. The program meets the needs of newly employed staff members as well as Level II fieldwork students.

CONCLUSION

The Splinting Assistance Program has been well received by new and experienced staff members and has been an enrichment experience for the Level II Fieldwork students. The Splinting Assistance Program has been an asset to the department's inservice education program and has promoted consistency in the quality of splints requested by specific physicians for treatment of their patients.

DISCUSSION

An experienced assistant with expertise in splinting developed a Splinting Assistance Program after receiving many requests for splinting information from therapists in other specialty areas as well as requests from new staff. The Splinting Assistance Program also serves as the assistant's special project in the department. The methods and procedures for development and organization of the workshops are described. This program orients all staff, especially new staff and Level II Fieldwork students to splinting techniques every quarter. The program has been in practice for a year and a half and continues because of staff needs.

REFERENCES

Cannon, N.M., Foltz, R.W., Koepfer, J.M., Lauck, M.F., Simpson, D.M., Bromley, R.S. (1985). *Manual of Hand Splinting*. New York: Churchill Livingstone.

Malick, M.H. (1976). *Manual on Static Hand Splinting*. Vol. 1. (2nd ed.). Pittsburgh: Harmerville Rehabilitation Center.

The Autosyringe Backpack for Children with Cancer: A Device that Permits Mobility

Debra Galvan Nordstrom, COTA

SUMMARY. A Certified Occupational Therapy Assistant, who was especially interested in the problems of the hospitalized pediatric oncology patient, describes an autosyringe backpack used during periods of chemotherapy administration. Use of the backpack permits greater mobility for the pediatric patient and enhances the ability of a child to accomplish physical, psychosocial and play development during periods of hospitalization. Construction information is included.

INTRODUCTION

This article describes an autosyringe backpack developed by a Certified Occupational Therapy Assistant (COTA) that allows mobility for the pediatric patient while also permitting him to perform developmental tasks during administration of chemotherapy treatment of cancer. The backpack provides independent mobility and increases the time a child can play and interact freely with others, thereby reducing the iatrogenic effects of hospitalization. Instructions for construction of the backpack are included.

Debra Galvan Nordstrom previously worked in the Pediatric Division of the Department of Occupational Therapy at the University of Texas Medical Branch, Galveston, TX 77550-2777. She is currently employed in the Health South Rehabilitation Hospital, Humble, TX 77338.

This article appears jointly in *Certified Occupational Therapy Assistants: Opportunities and Challenges* (The Haworth Press, 1988) and *Occupational Therapy in Health Care,* Volume 5, Numbers 2/3 (1988).

BACKGROUND

As a result of advancements in diagnosis and treatment of pediatric malignancies, a population of pediatric cancer survivors with very distinct psychological problems is rapidly developing. According to reports of the American Cancer Society, cancer is responsible for the largest number of deaths among U.S. children between the ages of three and fourteen. In 1960, a five-year survival rate was considered extremely rare. In contrast, the American Cancer Society now reports that the expected survival rate for children with acute lymphoblastic leukemias is now 50 % to 70 % of those who have undergone medical treatment. Many of these children who are treated in teaching hospitals or special facilities may have sequential admissions. This represents a significant change from the 1960 statistics (Brunnquell, 1982).

DEVELOPMENTAL NEEDS OF CHILDREN WITH CANCER

Children with cancer often have a variety of problems that require intervention beyond that provided by the family or through routine medical care. Upon admission to a hospital the child encounters strangers, unfamiliar settings, unpredictable events and painful, sometimes frightening medical procedures. For the chronically ill child, medical care involves giving up a degree of independence, especially in bodily matters, to the care and control of health care providers.

Present in almost every facet of illness and treatment of cancer are issues of control and competence. These issues are important for children because between infancy and adulthood their major developmental advancements are in the areas of greater self-control, interpersonal relationships, and environmental mastery. These developmental milestones are seriously threatened by cancer (Brunnquell, 1982).

During the preschool period, a sense of autonomy and self-control develops even when hospitalization places restrictions on usual childhood activities (Hobbs, 1985). When mobility is restricted, positive measures should be taken by occupational therapists to counteract the negative effects of hospitalization and other conditions caused by illness and to plan for the alleviation of unfavorable psychosocial factors (Willard & Spackman, 1947).

A major side effect of hospitalization is that of impaired mobility and activity (Brunnquell, 1982). This is often the case with oncology patients due to ongoing intravenous administration of medication, blood, or fluids, or bodily weakness, pain and nausea. A major form of restriction is administration of intravenous medication in the treatment of leukemia. All the above interrupt the child's patterns of activity. For example, one child with cancer at the University of Texas Medical Branch (UTMB) related that he despised remaining in his bed with the side rails up because he felt like a baby. Having to stay in a hospital room can lead significantly to a child's depression as a small room is not developmentally stimulating for the child (Brunnquell, 1980).

OCCUPATIONAL THERAPY GOALS FOR PEDIATRIC ONCOLOGY PATIENTS

Occupational therapy programs are concerned with the physical, psychosocial and vocational needs of individuals suffering with cancer. However, concern is not enough. Because the childhood cancer survivor rate has increased significantly since 1960, positive measures must be taken to assist these children in coping with their illness through the utilization of age appropriate activities. Children with cancer are entitled to the same opportunities to explore their environment in the quest for attainment of developmental skills, as is any other child. Occupational therapy goals in an oncology program may include the building of self-esteem, the reduction of anxiety and depression and the promotion of usefulness through age appropriate activities. According to Oelrich (1974), "activity that is consistent with the patient's physical potential serves to prevent undue regression and promotes self-esteem." Pediatric occupational therapists can assist the young patient in discovering or rediscovering deprived childhood activities which are restricted or forbidden by the rigors of cancer routines and hospitalization.

DEVELOPMENT OF THE AUTOSYRINGE BACKPACK

After observing children either remaining in their rooms or having to rely on others to assist them in fulfilling their developmental needs, a solution to permit mobility was sought by the occupational therapy staff in pediatrics. The solution had to be one that avoided placing the child in a position to be taunted by hospital peers and one that was effective in permitting independent mobility and activity while receiving medication.

Some chemotherapy medications such as ARA-C and Adrimycin can be infused through a device called an autosyringe. The autosyringe allows small volumes of chemotherapy to be infused over a prolonged period of time. This form of administration is preferred over the conventional intravenous (I.V.) drip because the autosyringe (Figure 1) is able to infuse 3-10ccs per hour whereas the I.V. pumps cannot infuse such small volumes without loss of accuracy. Traditionally the conventional intravenous drip unit was attached to an I.V. pole with casters (Figure 2). This permitted some mobility for a child during the administration of chemotherapy because a parent or health care worker could move the pole and allow

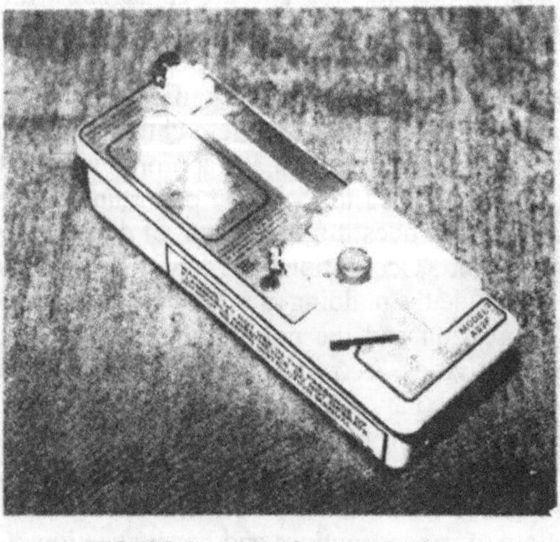

FIGURE 1. Autosyringe mechanism

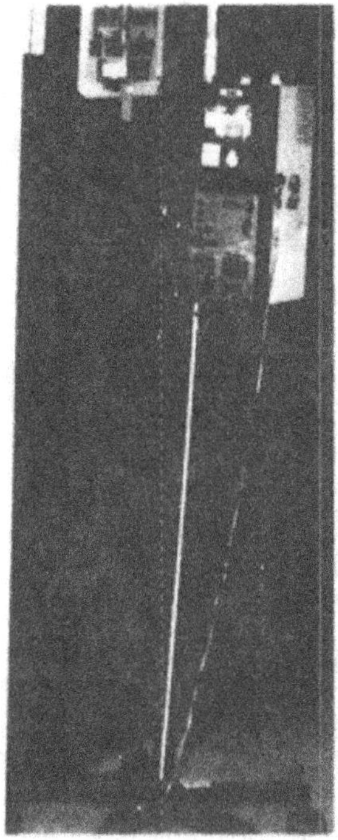

FIGURE 2. Pole with rollers with I.V. monitor attached

the child some measure of freedom of movement. After the autosyringe was introduced to the oncology unit it was not possible to attach it to the usual I.V. pole. When the autosyringe needle was placed subcutaneously in the child's arm and secured, so that usual movement did not dislodge it, the child had to remain in bed during the administration of the chemotherapy.

After exploring the limitations of the autosyringe mechanism and re-examining the goal of providing independent mobility for the child, the COTA on the pediatric service developed a backpack (Figure 3) for the autosyringe mechanism (see Figure 4.)

The COTA was especially interested in the problems of the pediatric oncology patients. She participated in community and parent support groups such as The Candlelighters and The Rainbow Connection, and accompanied the children on special summer camp experiences. Even when the COTA was transferred to another ser-

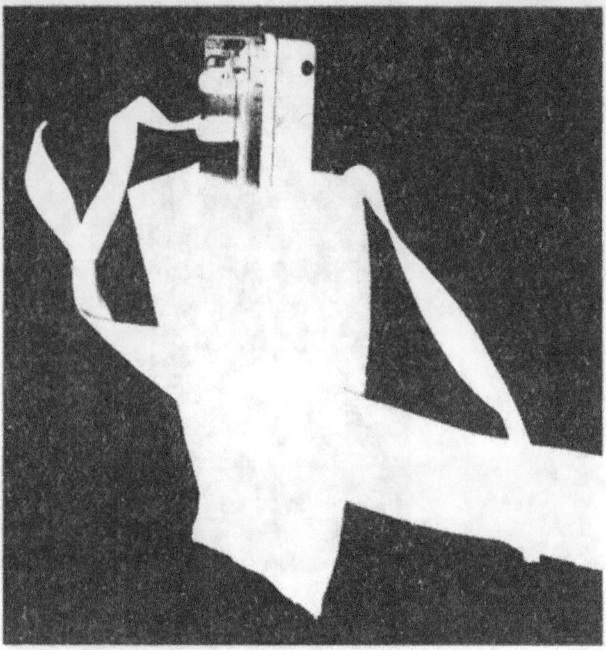

FIGURE 3. Autosyringe in backpack

vice in the department, she retained her responsibilities on the pediatric oncology service.

Developmentally the autosyringe backpack is a valuable device to augment a child's development in any occupational therapy pediatric oncology program. The backpack can help alleviate "cabin fever," permit the child some control in his environment, maintain and increase the child's self-esteem, and serve as a validation of ability.

CONCLUSION

The autosyringe backpack has been instrumental in permitting the oncology patient to successfully explore the environment, interact with peers, and attain normal developmental milestones. The autosyringe backpack has good patient compliance because back-

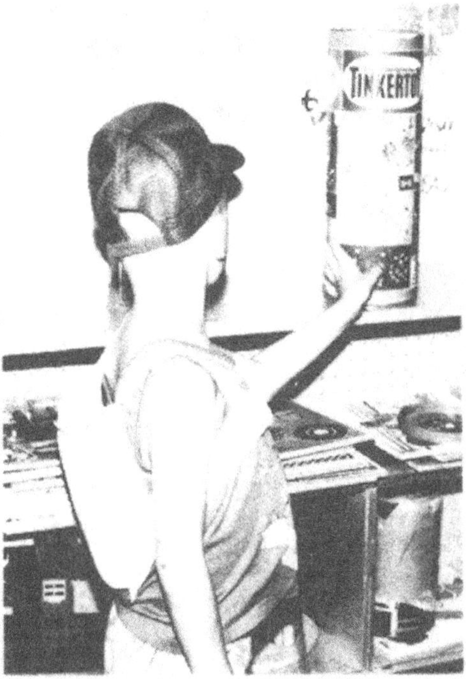

FIGURE 4. Child wearing autosyringe backpack (demonstration only; infusion needle is not inserted)

packs are popular with school children and are much used by medical students to carry belongings in the child's hospital environment.

The backpack concept is appreciated by the pediatricians at UTMB over other methods because the autosyringe is placed behind the child's back, thus keeping it out of sight. With the autosyringe out of the child's line of vision, the potential of the child to tamper with the unit is diminished.

DISCUSSION

The percentage of survival rates for children with leukemia has improved since 1960. When hospitalized, these children need to experience age appropriate developmental activities. Usual methods of chemotherapy administration restrict the child's mobility and activity. A COTA reports the development of a backpack holder for the autosyringe that allows a child to have general mobility while chemotherapy is being administered. The device has been well accepted by pediatricians and patients. Instructions for fabrication of the autosyringe backpack are contained in the Appendix.

REFERENCES

Brunnquell, D., Hall, M.D. (1982). Issues in the psychological care of pediatric oncology patients. *American Journal of Orthopsychiatry*, *52*(1), 32-44.

Hobbs, N., Perrin, J.M., Ireys, H.T. (1985). *Chronic illness and the family*. San Francisco: Josey-Bass.

Oelrich, M. (1974). The patient with a fatal illness. *American Journal of Occupational Therapy*, *28*, 429-432.

Willard, H.S., Spackman, C.B. (1947). *Occupational therapy*. Philadelphia: J.B. Lippincott.

APPENDIX: BACKPACK CONSTRUCTION

Backpack Materials

2 inch webbing
1 inch webbing
Flannel Duck Fabric
  Panel A 9 inches × 6 inches
  Panel B 9 inches × 9 1/2 inches
3 inches of 2 inch loop and hook Velcro
1 inch of 1 inch hook Velcro
2 inches of 1 inch loop Velcro

Measurements/Cutting

1. Measure circumference of child's chest under arms and one inch below nipples and add 3 inches to chest measurement.
2. Cut two pieces of flannel duck as indicated above.
3. Cut 1 chest strap of 2 inch webbing the length, plus three inches, of the chest measurement.

4. Cut 2 shoulder straps from 1 inch webbing according to instruction 13 under Fabrication.

Fabrication

1. Place chest strap flat on table. Place the 2 inch loop Velcro on top of the left end of the chest strap. Sew Velcro in place.
2. Turn the chest strap over. The right end now becomes the left end and the left end becomes the right. Sew the 3 inch piece of the hook Velcro on the left end of the chest strap.
3. With the loop Velcro facing upward, mark the middle of the chest strap by folding the two ends of the chest strap vertically and horizontally.
4. Sew the end of the 2 inch loop Velcro to the middle of the top edge of backpack Panel A.
5. Sew lengthwise, the 1 inch hook Velcro to the middle top edge of backpack Panel B.
6. Find the middle of the backpack Panel A by folding lengthwise and widthwise. Mark the center with a dot.
7. With flannel side up, match the dots on the chest strap, and backpack panel A.
8. Sew chest strap of the two inch webbing to Panel A.
9. Turn strap over where the hook Velcro is on the left facing upward.
10. Panel B is wider than Panel A to allow for tucks. With flannel side up, pin Panel B to Panel A leaving top and bottom open. Make tucks at bottom and fold outward, and pin.
11. Sew tucks with a straight stitch 1/4 inch from bottom edge.
12. Sew Panel A and Panel B together along side and bottom, using a zig zag stitch to prevent fraying.
13. To measure for fitting of the shoulder straps, place chest strap with backpack in the middle of the child's back, and fasten with Velcro in front. The top of the pack should be in line with the top of the scapulae. Measure the shoulder straps, which should rest in the middle of the shoulder. Allow one half inch on each strap for sewing.
14. Sew one shoulder strap on the outside of the chest strap in front and inside of backpack at the child's back.

15. Repeat for the other shoulder strap.
16. When the I.V. needle has been placed and attached to the autosyringe, the autosyringe can be placed in the back pack which has been placed on the child and fastened with the two inch Velcro. (See Figure 4.)

Toy Adaptations in Pediatrics

Elaine Lemire, COTA

SUMMARY. This report describes a special project of a Certified Occupational Therapy Assistant on a pediatric rehabilitation unit who learned to adapt battery operated toys for use by multihandicapped children. This led to the enhancement of patient treatment and requests for the assistant to consult with other professionals. Instructions are given for fabricating simple controls for use by handicapped children to activate battery operated toys.

INTRODUCTION

This article will describe a Special Project (Clakeley, 1988) which the author, a Certified Occupational Therapy Assistant (COTA), developed on a Pediatric Rehabilitation Unit. The project resulted in new learning that led to enhancement of patient treatment through adaptation of battery operated toys so that severely handicapped children could activate them. This learning was used to plan and conduct a hands-on workshop to teach other professionals how to adapt the toys. Since then, the assistant's consultation has been sought to advise other professionals on selection and adaptation of toys.

Elaine Lemire works in the Pediatric Rehabilitation Service and Occupational Therapy Department of the University of Texas Medical Branch Hospitals, Galveston, TX 77550-2777. She graduated from Galveston Community College and has a Certificate of Proficiency in Occupational Therapy from the School of Allied Health Sciences of University of Texas Medical Branch.

This article appears jointly in *Certified Occupational Therapy Assistants: Opportunities and Challenges* (The Haworth Press, 1988) and *Occupational Therapy in Health Care,* Volume 5, Numbers 2/3 (1988).

BACKGROUND

The COTA works with severely handicapped cerebral palsied children, children with developmental delays, and children in the rehabilitation phase following extensive severe burns. Childrens' play and its importance to learning, cognitive development, and occupational choice have been well described by occupational therapists (Florey, Matsutsuyu, Maurer, Michelman & Takata, 1971). The severely physically handicapped child may not have motor skills that enable him to participate fully in play (Gralewicz, 1973).

When children have difficulty with normal play and motor movements, toys can be a great motivator for encouraging them to respond. Battery activated toys are a source of pleasure for children to watch. However, this is a passive activity, whereas the ability to switch toys on or off gives the child more control of the toys and the environment. However, most battery operated toys have small or concealed switches that prevent handicapped children from being independent in play with such toys.

SPECIAL PROJECT

Three events occurred that led to the development of a special project to adapt battery operated toys for the multihandicapped child. First, a co-worker loaned the COTA a copy of Linda Burkhart's book (1982), which contained instructions for using (1) materials usually found in an occupational therapy clinic and (2) wire to adapt simple switches for toys. Second, the unit received a Special Education Grant designated for purchasing equipment and for parent education. Third, some of the funds allocated to occupational therapy were used to purchase toys, and with the information from the Burkhart book (1982), the COTA's task was to adapt them for the childrens' use.

The book provided instruction for soldering and wiring, but because its directions were not totally clear, some trial and error learning and problem solving were necessary. After practicing these beginning tasks it was then possible to construct a simple switch.

The supervisor allocated time for shopping for toys and this was done using some of the guidelines in the book for purchase of toys and adapting them. Recommended toys and others the COTA thought could be adapted were purchased.

The goal was to adapt a switch or control that would enable the child to activate the toy by turning the power source (batteries) on or off. A common solution to this problem is a large area flap switch (Shein & Mandell, 1982) that can be activated by minimal pressure and be positioned so that any part of the child's body can be used to turn the adapted toy's switch on.

Toys are a marvelous motivator for children and battery operated toys with any kind of control make it possible for the child to not only play with a toy but also to have some control over the environment. This is a special need for children who because of illness or injury may not have the ability to perform fine motor operations and can benefit from some kind of switch control toy.

Burkhardt's (1982) guidelines for toys suggested the use of battery operated toys that move, make sounds, or perform some simple activity, such as drumming (see Figure 1), as being the best for adaptation. Also recommended were toys that do not move out of the child's control. A few mistakes were made such as adapting a robot whose wire moved it out of the range within which the child could control its return to him, thus depriving the child of independence in operating it. If a child cannot move about, such as on a mat, then it is not beneficial to adapt a toy that requires its return to the child by someone else. Another questionable purchase was a toy vehicle with a loud siren. The children loved it but the staff found the sound too loud for comfort.

The amount of pressure needed to activate the switch, which can be adjusted, should be taken into consideration for a given patient. For example, a child with burns claimed he was not able to touch anything, but he would play for long periods using a soft foam covered pressure switch to activate a toy.

For those children who are unable to perform fine motor movements to play with toys, the adaptation of battery powered toys that move, make sounds or perform are the best choice for adaptation. Simple switches that can be activated with any moving body part can be made to motivate the child to use a movement or a position that is part of the treatment plan. While performing the movement, the toy is activated as a reward.

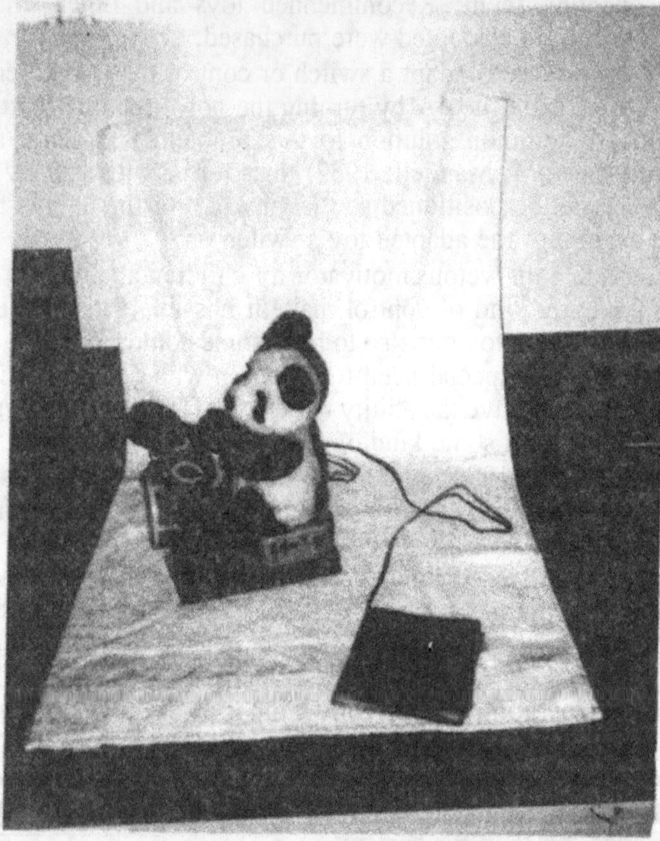

FIGURE 1. Adapted Drummer Bear. Flat switch in lower right corner connected. The circuit breaker (jack) is inserted in the switch at left rear side of the bear.

The pressure control switches or large area flap switches have been very useful because of simplicity of fabrication. More importantly, the child can activate the switch with any body part that can move against the switch. Use of these child activated toys has resulted in improved head control and weight bearing for some patients. Neurodevelopmental treatment (NDT) is often used on our unit, and use of adapted toys can be incorporated into some of those activities by having the activation of a toy or sound be the end product of the NDT sequence planned by the therapist (Anderson, Hinojosa & Stauch, 1987).

WORKSHOP

The next assignment on this project was to conduct a workshop to demonstrate methods for adapting toys to other therapists, parents and teachers. The attendees made one switch before leaving (see Appendix). Eleven attended the workshop, and the evaluation forms indicated its success because the attendees liked the hands-on opportunity and completing a switch to take home.

The assistant learned that the workshop would have gone more smoothly if the procedures for each component of constructing a switch had been at separate work stations, with a skilled person at each work station to demonstrate and guide the participants through.

DISCUSSION

The work with adapted toys has added a new dimension to the assistant's job. She sees a wider variety of children than might ordinarily have been referred and is asked to consult on types of toys and kinds of switches that can be adapted for them. Also, other therapists have called for advice about completing projects with adapted switches. Physical therapists and speech therapists have consulted with her about design of adapted switches for their patients, and information on adaptation of toys was presented at a Texas Medical Association meeting.

The trial and error experiences with wiring and adapting toys have been very useful in learning how to trouble shoot and problem solve, leading to decisions on types of switches for varying needs. Since beginning the project and learning methods and procedures for adapting controls, the assistant has discovered another book (Wright & Nomura, 1985), which has made it possible to learn how to adapt computer controls for multihandicapped children to facilitate communication.

CONCLUSION

This report indicated methods to choose and adapt battery operated toys for use by multihandicapped children. Resources for instruction and trial and error learning resulted in successful adaptation of the toys. Guidelines for toy selection are included. The use of adapted toys has resulted in improved head control and weight bearing for some patients. The assistant has experienced and expanded new dimensions in her work because she receives consultations to help a wider variety of children through the use of the adapted toys.

REFERENCES

Anderson, J., Hinojosa, J. and Strauch, C. (1987). Integrating play in neurodevelopmental treatment. *American Journal of Occupational Therapy, 41*(7), 421-426.

Burkhart, L. J. (1982). *More homemade battery devices for severely handicapped children with suggested activities*. College Park, MD: Burkhart Publisher (8315 Potomac Avenue).

Clakeley, G. L. (1988). Designing job enrichment projects. Occupational Therapy in Health Care, *5*(2/3), 47-53.

D'Aloisio, S. (1987). Special toys educate children with learning disabilities. *OT Week*, *1*(22), 12-13. Rockville, MD: The American Occupational Therapy Association.

Florey, L. (1971). An approach to play and play development. *American Journal of Occupational Therapy*, *25*(6), 275-280.

Gralewicz, A. (1973). Play deprivation in multihandicapped children. *American Journal of Occupational Therapy*, *27*(2), 70-72.

Matsutsuyu, J. (1971). Occupational behavior – a perspective on work and play. *American Journal of Occupational Therapy*, *25*(6), 291-294.

Maurer, P. (1971). Antecedents of work behavior. *American Journal of Occupational Therapy*, *25*(6), 295-297.

Michelman, S. (1971). The importance of creative play. *American Journal of Occupational Therapy*, *25*(6), 285-290.

Shein, G. F., and Mandel, A. R. (1982). Large area flap switch to control battery-operated toys. *American Journal of Occupational Therapy*, *36*(2), 107-110.

Takata, N. (1971). The play milieu – a preliminary appraisal. *American Journal of Occupational Therapy*, *25*(6), 281-284.

Wright, D. Nomura, M. (1985). *From toys to computers*. San Jose, CA: Wright, Nomura Publishers. P.O. Box 700242, San Jose, CA 95170.

RESOURCES

Flaghouse, Inc. *Special Populations, Catalogue*, 18 W. 18th St. New York, NY 10011. (212) 989-9700. Sells toys, movement and positioning aids, devices for computer access.

Handicapped Childrens Technological Services, Inc., P.O. Box 7, Foster, RI 02825. Sells a variety of modified battery powered toys.

Steven Kanor, PhD, Toy Adaptor. 8 Main Street, Hastings On Hudson, NY 10706. (914) 478-0960.

Stanford Rehabilitation Engineering, Children's Hospital at Stanford, 520 Willow Road, Palo Alto, CA 94303. Can make custom switches, sells toy adapters, latching interface boxes and modifies existing switches.

The Able Child, 325 W. 11th Street, New York, NY 10014. Sells a variety of adapted and standard toys.

Toys for Special Children, 101 Lefurgy Avenue, Hastings On Hudson, NY 10706 (914) 478-0960. Sells adapters and a variety of adapted toys including popular wind-up toys which operate on a single switch.

Zygo Industries, Inc., P.O. Box 108, Portland OR 97207-1008. Sells adapters, adapted toys. A good selection of commonly used switches and a mounting kit for switch attachment. They also have devices for non-oral communication and computer access.

APPENDIX: INSTRUCTIONS FOR ADAPTING BATTERY OPERATED TOYS

Guides for Decisions on Toys to Adapt

1. Which method will work? (Copper wafer or permanent jack?) If the toy can open with access to on/off switch, it is possible to use a jack. It will be necessary to drill a hole in the toy at the switch to mount the jack. If the toy cannot be opened, it will be necessary to use a copper wafer to adapt the toy.
2. If the copper wafer is selected, the toy should have only an on/off switch.
3. Battery box should be easily accessible and have plenty of room.
4. If the toy is one that moves, such as a jeep or robot, the child will need assistance when the toy moves to the end of the wire.
5. Is there more than one way to use the toy?

Tools/Supplies for Adapting Toys

Tools

1. Soldering iron with safe support stand. (25-30 watt is enough power for these tasks)
2. Utility knife
3. Wire stripper
4. Heavy duty scissors
5. Vise to hold objects while working
6. Leather punch.

Supplies

1. Thin rosin core solder
2. 24 or 22 gauge stranded speaker wire
3. Electrical or masking tape
4. Double stick carpet tape
5. Poster board
6. Disposable aluminum cookie sheets or pans
7. Foam rubber 1/4″ thick

8. Copper clad board, or copper foil (used for tooling)
9. Plugs and jacks. Either 1/16″ subminiature size or 1/8″ miniature. The trend in commercially available toys and switches is toward 1/8″. However, most tape recorders require 1/16″ subminiature size. These are available from Radio Shack Stores.

Soldering Tips

1. Wires and terminals must be clean to solder. Use steel wool to clean the wires and terminals.
2. Be sure the soldering iron is hot. It is preferable to use a soldering iron that has a holder to protect you and the work surface from damage.
3. Thread wires though holes in terminals and twist them around themselves separately. When soldering two wires to the same part, twist the wires together.
4. Touch solder to the soldering iron briefly, then touch soldering iron to parts being soldered together.
5. Pliers or vices are helpful in holding parts together while soldering. (*Helping Hands* from Radio Shack are great for this.)
6. Be careful when using soldering irons—they get very hot. Be sure to unplug the soldering iron when it is not in use.

Circuit Breaker

Materials

6″ piece of speaker wire
1/8″ miniature phone plug
2 pieces of copper foil 5/8″ × 1″
4 pieces 1/2″ electrical tape 3/4″ long
1 piece double stick tape 5/8″ × 1″

Fabrication

1. Cut 1″ slit in the plastic between two strands of speaker wire. Spread apart and use wire stripper to remove plastic from last 1/2″ of wire.
2. Fasten each piece of stripped wire to a 1/8″ shielded phone plug. There are two pieces of metal on the plug with the hole.

Place one wire through each hole and bend wire back on itself and twist around. Solder wire in place. Do not move curved piece of metal because it forms contact with the plug from the switch pad. Wrap one piece of electrical tape around each wire to prevent the two stands from making contact with each other.

3. Repeat step 1 above to the other end of the speaker wire.
4. Solder one wire to the 5/8″ by 1″ piece of copper foil.
5. Solder second wire to second 5/8″ × 1″ piece of copper foil.
6. Wrap one piece of electrical tape around any exposed wire not soldered to foil.
7. Remove backing from carpet tape and place it on one side of copper foil that does not have the soldered wire on it. Remove other backing from tape and place second piece of copper foil without solder on tape and press two pieces of copper together. The two pieces of copper must not touch each other.

This circuit breaker can be used by placing the copper strip between the battery in the toy and the positive terminal, and then closing the cover of the battery box. If there are two batteries, it is necessary to insert the circuit breaker on one. To activate the toy, insert 1/8″ plug from large area switch into 1/8″ jack.

Secure the jack to the outside of the toy with tape. It may be necessary to tape the battery compartment closed. When the circuit breaker is in place, the toy switch should be in the ON position or it will not operate from the large area flat switch.

Large Area Flat Switch

Tools

1. Soldering iron
2. Vice to hold pieces together
3. Heavy duty scissors
4. Wire stripper
5. Leather punch

Supplies

2 squares 6″ × 6″ cut from disposable aluminum cookie sheet
2 squares 6″ × 6″ cut from poster board
4 cubes of 1/4″ foam (1/4″ × 1/4″ × 1/4″)
Double stick carpet tape: 2 pieces 6″ × 6″, and 8 1/4″ squares
Speaker wire long enough to reach from switch to toy (The two strands of speaker wire are protected from each other by a plastic covering.)
1/8″ miniature phone jack

Construction of Switch

1. Punch hole in each piece of aluminum with leather punch. A hole should be in upper right corner of one piece and upper left corner of the other.
2. Strip plastic for 1/2″ from one end of speaker wire. This will leave two ends of stripped wire.
3. Place one stripped wire through hole in aluminum, bend over and twist to itself. Repeat on other piece of aluminum.
4. Remove protective backing from one side of 6″ square of double stick carpet tape. Apply to one side of aluminum square. Remove the other protective backing and apply poster board to it. Repeat for second pair of 6″ squares of aluminum and poster board.
5. Remove backing from one side of the 1/4″ square of double sided carpet tape. Apply to one side of 1/4″ foam cube. Turn over and place foam cube on a corner of the 6″ square. Repeat this step for other three corners of the 6″ square. Remove double stick tape and place on top of each of the four foam cubes. Remove the second backing and place the second aluminum square over the four foam cubes and carefully line up the sides evenly.
6. Split and strip the other end of the wire and solder to 1/8″ miniature phone jack.

The miniature phone jack is placed into the miniature phone plug on the circuit breaker.

Occupational Therapy and Low Vision Rehabilitation

Terri L. Reichley, COTA

SUMMARY. This article addresses low vision rehabilitation programs and the certified occupational therapy assistant's role in a low vision, outpatient, ambulatory-care service. An individual who acquires low vision secondary to eye or brain pathology may have some useful vision but not enough to facilitate ease in performing activities of daily living. Visual tasks, such as reading, writing, homemaking and leisure activities become quite difficult without medical and therapeutic intervention. In these instances, the efforts of eye care professionals and occupational therapists can be coordinated to provide a holistic approach to patient treatment. The primary objective in utilizing a low vision rehabilitation program is to provide instruction to patients with low vision problems in activities of daily living through the use of optical/nonoptical aids to achieve functional independence.

A major objective in occupational therapy is to facilitate the restoration and maintenance of independence for individuals whose

---

Terri L. Reichley is a 1985 honor graduate of Mount Aloysius Junior College. She has been employed as Certified Occupational Therapy Assistant in the Occupational Therapy Department of Geisinger Medical Center, Danville, PA. For further information contact Ms. Reichley through the Department of Physical Medicine and Rehabilitation 01-48, Geisinger Medical Center, Danville, PA 17822.

The author gratefully acknowledges Judith L. Bianchi, OD, and Thomas J. Ciucci, OTR/L, whose efforts and support allowed her to develop a low vision rehabilitation program at Geisinger.

All photographs in this paper are by Nathan N. Jeffery.

This article appears jointly in *Certified Occupational Therapy Assistants: Opportunities and Challenges* (The Haworth Press, 1988) and *Occupational Therapy in Health Care*, Volume 5, Numbers 2/3 (1988).

level of function in activities of daily life has been physically and/or emotionally impaired. When an individual acquires *low vision* secondary to an eye or brain pathology, a decrease in function and a resultant loss of independence is often experienced to some degree. Activities of daily living (A.D.L.) such as reading, writing, homemaking and leisure activities become quite difficult without medical and therapeutic intervention. At Geisinger Medical Center in Danville, Pennsylvania, the efforts of an optometrist and a certified occupational therapy assistant (COTA) are being coordinated to provide a comprehensive outpatient program of evaluation, education and instruction for low vision patients.

LOW VISION AND THE REHABILITATION SERVICE

Vision rehabilitation is a newly emerging area of expertise in occupational therapy. The low vision rehabilitation service is designed to help those with constricted fields of view and/or those with decreased visual acuity to compensate for and adapt to the results of their sight impairment, to function at an optimum level and to live a self-sufficient lifestyle (Jose, 1985). This philosophy seems to parallel that of the occupational therapy profession and correlates with the traditional role which occupational therapists can play in fostering functional independence.

In order to better understand the need for such a service, one must examine the meaning of low vision and the functional implications which may result. Simply stated, low vision is located in the middle of a spectrum between "normal" vision and "blindness" (Colenbrander, 1976). Those with low vision have lower than normal vision, but do have some remaining sight which they can be taught to use to the fullest potential (Colenbrander, 1976). According to Faye (1976), "Loss of vision may be caused by systemic disease, acute or chronic diseases localized in the eye, or a birth defect involving the visual apparatus" (p. 7). Low vision can affect the performance of a college student who is unable to read the blackboard or an elderly gentleman who can no longer see to plant seeds in his garden. Fortunately, there is help for these individuals. Rehabilitation encompasses vocational, educational and leisure skills with the emphasis of treatment centering on the needs and objectives of the patient (Jose, 1985). An interdisciplinary team of professionals can work with low vision patients to ". . . enhance their level of visual activity" (Jose, 1985, p. 62) and their independence with A.D.L. skills.

At Geisinger the individual with low vision must first have a visual/ocular health examination performed by an ophthalmologist or an optometrist to determine appropriateness for low vision services. If the person is found to be a candidate, a referral is made to the Low Vision Specialist—an optometrist—whose examination combines a medical history with the diagnostic examination which leads to prescription of optical/nonoptical visual aids. After determining the need for an aid(s), the Low Vision Specialist refers the patient to Occupational Therapy. In this setting the COTA performs an A.D.L.-type evaluation which results in training in such areas as adaptation of the physical environment, compensation for visual disturbance and proper use of the visual aid(s).

TRAINING WITH LOW VISION AIDS

A visual aid is "a device that can magnify, filter, or increase the usable field of vision" (Cockerham, 1984, p. 14). Mellor (1986) stated "There are lenses for close work, for intermediate range, for distance viewing" (p. 24). A widely held misconception is that low vision aids have a direct affect on the user's eye pathology. In actuality, low vision aids do not affect the health of the eye, cause the disease process to get better or worse, or cure or restore the patient's eyesight (Hollander, 1981). They do, however, enable the user to perform activities of daily life which were previously difficult.

Visual aids may be ". . . optical lenses such as magnifiers or (microscopes), telescopes, or non-optical devices . . ." (Hollander, 1981, p. 5) such as gooseneck lamps, felt-tip pens, large print watches or clocks, bold-lined checks, envelope guides and many others which can serve as therapeutic modalities in occupational therapy. Microscopes (see Figures 1 and 2) are often prescribed for activities which are performed at arm's length or closer. These activities are classified as near tasks and include, but are not limited

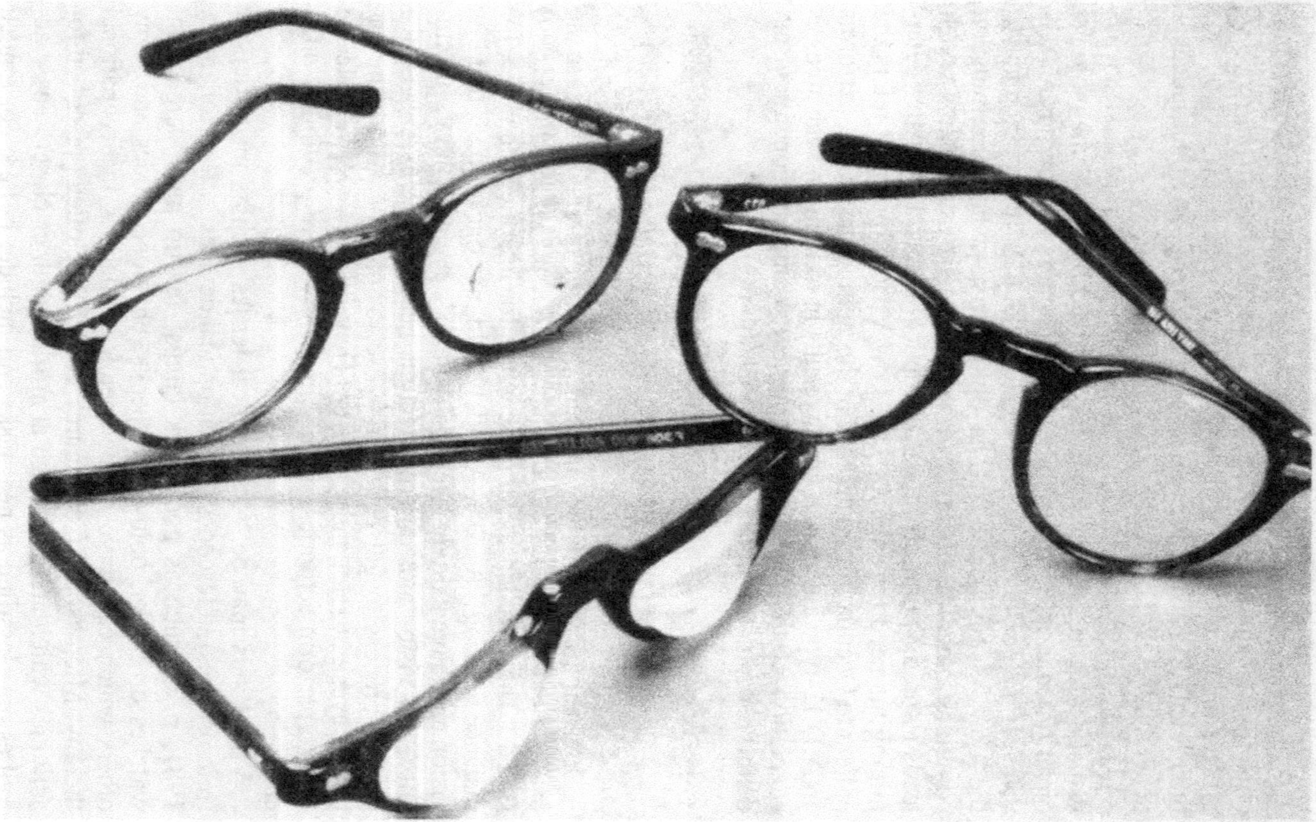

FIGURE 1. Spectacle—mounted microscopes—fullfield and half-eyes

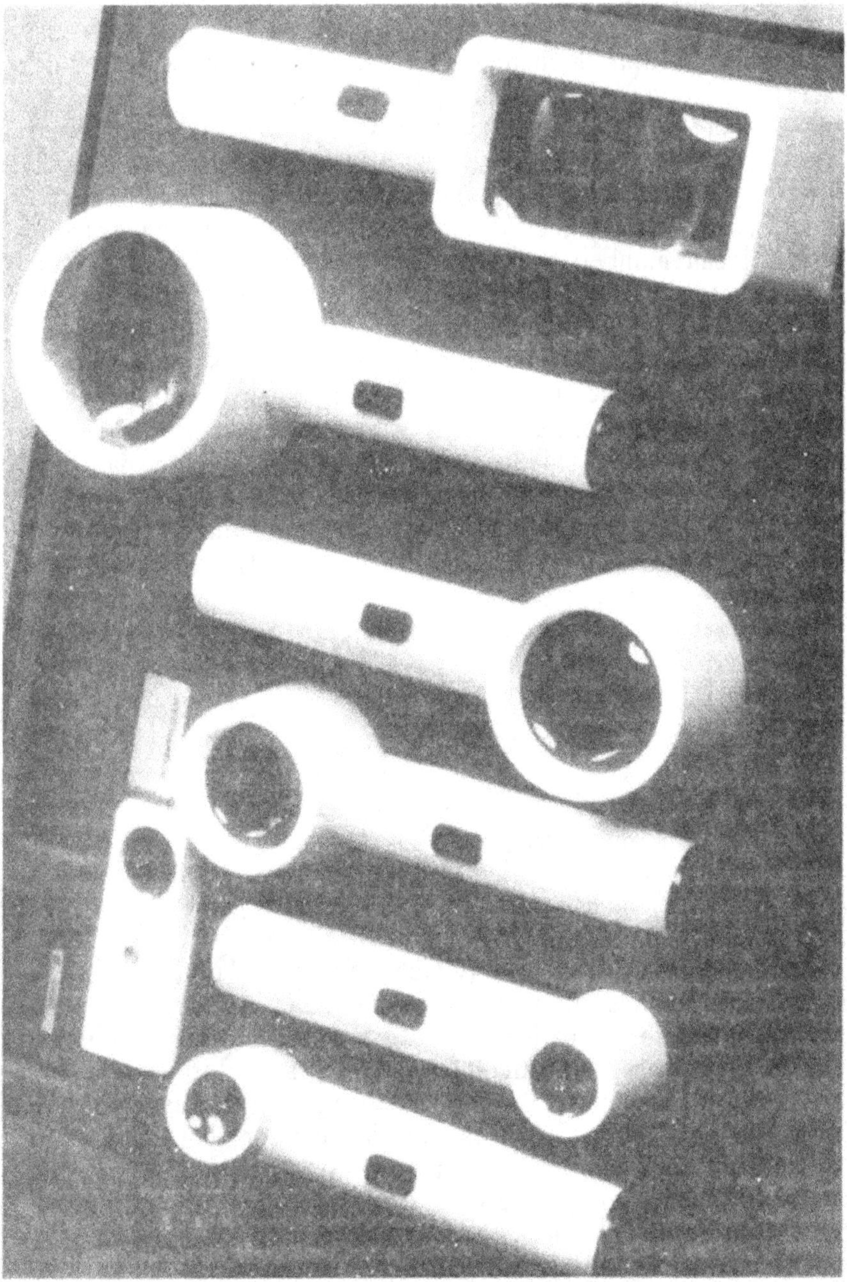

FIGURE 2. Hand-held, illuminated microscopes

to, reading, writing, homemaking tasks, management skills, leisure activities and vocational tasks (see Figure 3).

Telescopes (see Figure 4) are prescribed to facilitate distance viewing which includes those activities performed beyond arm's length. With a telescope, a low vision patient may view television, interpret words and objects on signs, read information from a chalkboard, locate numbers on doors or buses, identify persons within a large area and perform many other tasks (see Figure 5).

The COTA can provide education about the name, purpose, care, and maintenance of low vision aids. Training is also necessary so that the patient can learn ". . . to develop new patterns of coordinating movement of eye, head and body to compensate for distortions produced by the aid" (Mellor, 1986, p. 24). Increasing the patient's awareness of the various nonoptical aids (refer to Figure 3) which provide physical comfort, assist with self-care skills and enhance independence is another responsibility of the COTA.

CASE HISTORIES

The following cases provide an illustration of the need for and effectiveness of low vision rehabilitation. Mr. L.V. is an 84-year-old male with low vision who lives alone and who must be able to function independently. He was referred for low vision services, and the use of a microscope was prescribed. The patient's goals included developing the ability to independently read the newspaper and his mail, sign checks, and plant seeds in his garden.

During occupational therapy a gooseneck lamp (which increases illumination), an acetate filter (which, when placed over the surface of the reading material increases contrast), and a check guide were recommended for the patient. Training was also provided in the use of the microscope. A horticulture activity was performed with instructions for proper use of the microscope during this task. Suggestions regarding adaptation of the physical environment to facilitate gardening were also made. After two sessions of low vision training in occupational therapy, the individual successfully met all of his goals and resumed an independent life-style.

Ms. L.V. is a 30-year-old diabetic patient with low vision. Her primary responsibilities included caring for her husband and infant,

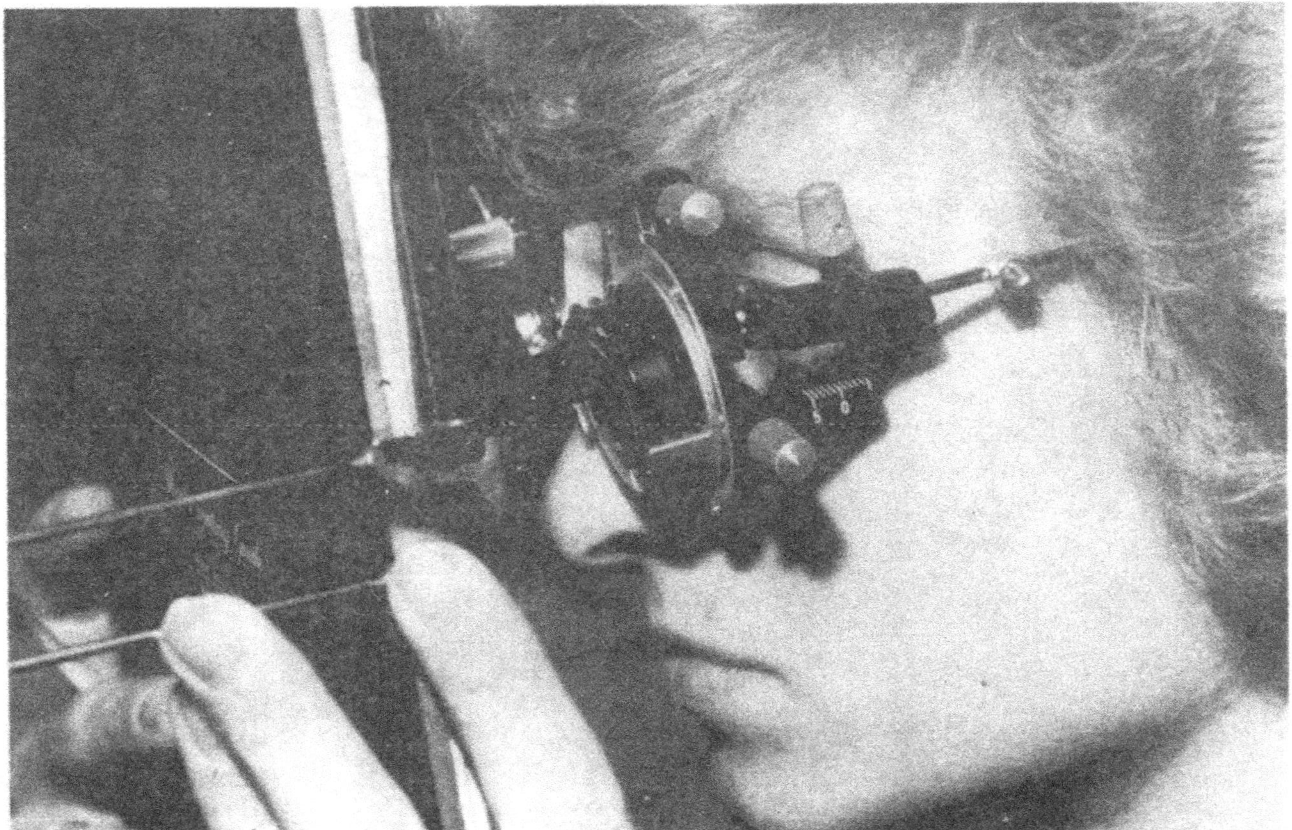

FIGURE 3. Individual wears trial frames containing a microscopic lens while reading material on a clipboard. The clipboard with extending line guide serves as a nonoptical aid to facilitate reading.

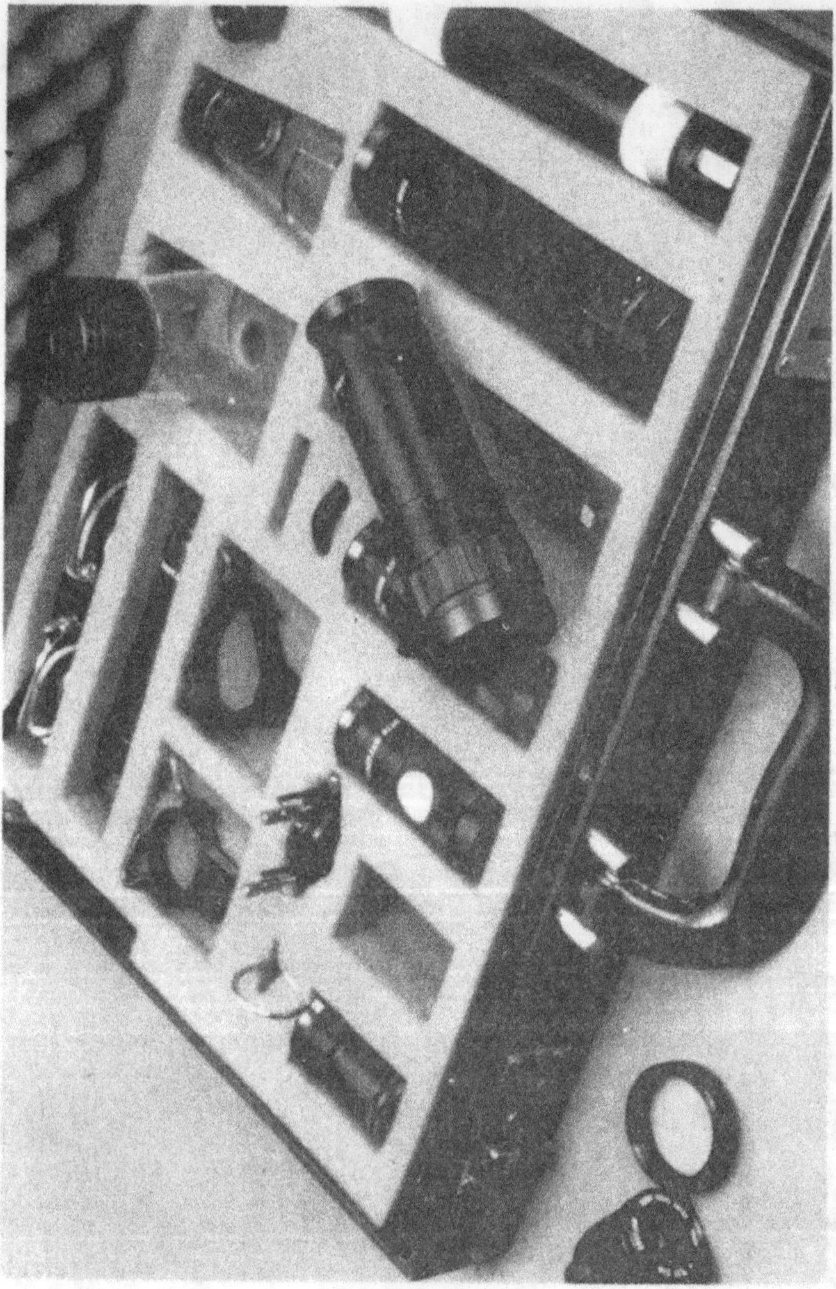

FIGURE 4. Various telescopes which can be spectacle-mounted or hand-held.

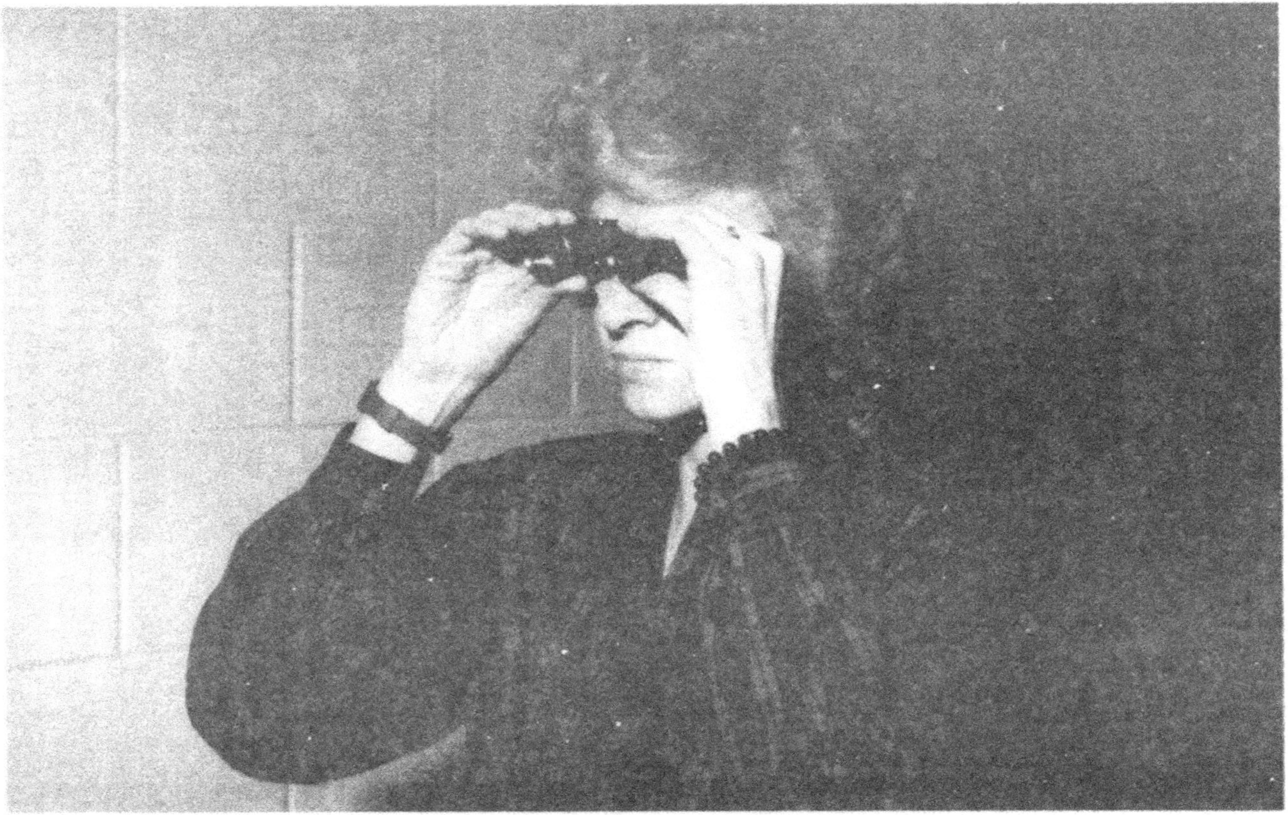

FIGURE 5. Individual focuses a telescope for distance viewing.

fulfilling most homemaking tasks and self-care, which involves administering her own insulin shots. L.V.'s personal goals included the ability to independently read storybooks to her child, to identify markings/temperatures on the stove dials, to recognize numbers on the syringe of the insulin needle, and to recognize street signs/highway markers. Near and distance training was provided by the COTA, using a microscope and a telescope in simulated situations to meet the patient's needs. The COTA also recommended that fluorescent orange markings be placed on the patient's stove dials to increase independence in the kitchen. The patient learned proper techniques when working with the aids, attained a level of functional independence and met all objectives.

CONCLUSION

A person with low vision becomes ". . . a candidate for rehabilitation when a visual disorder and/or impairment interferes with his or her ability to function . . ." (Gordon, 1976, p. 129). The COTA can plan an important part in facilitating the restoration of independence. Vision rehabilitation has proven to be very effective in this outpatient setting and has potential for private practice, as well.

REFERENCES

Cockerham, P. (Ed.). (1984). *Low Vision Questions and Answers: Definitions, Aids, Services* (pamphlet). New York: American Foundation for the Blind.

Colenbrander, A. (1976). Low vision: Definition and classification. In E. E. Faye's *Clinical Low Vision* (pp. 3-6). Boston: Little, Brown and Company, Inc.

Faye, E. E. (1976). Clinical definition and classification of the low vision patient. In E. E. Faye's *Clinical Low Vision* (pp. 7-13). Boston: Little, Brown and Company, Inc.

Gordon, A. R. (1976). Indications for rehabilitation for the low vision patient. In E. E. Faye's *Clinical Low Vision* (pp. 129-132). Boston: Little, Brown and Company, Inc.

Hollander, C. S. (1981). *Patient's Guide to Vision Rehabilitation for the Partially Sighted* (pamphlet). New York: Sight Improvement Center, Inc.

Jose, R. T. (Ed.). (1985). *Understanding Low Vision* (2nd printing). New York: American Foundation for the Blind.

Mellor, C. M. (1986). *Aids for the 80s – What They Are and What They Do* (5th printing). New York: American Foundation for the Blind.

SUGGESTED READING MATERIAL

In addition to the references previously listed, I have found the following material to be very beneficial in broadening my understanding of vision impairment and the importance of rehabilitation in this area.

Beliveau, M. & Smith, A. (Eds.). (1980, August). *The Interdisciplinary Approach to Low Vision Rehabilitation*. Prepared for the National Training Workshop in Low Vision. Co-sponsored by The American Foundation for the Blind, and The Rehabilitation Services Administration, Division of Manpower Development, Chicago.

Dickman, I. R. (1985). *Making Life More Livable* (2nd printing). New York: American Foundation for the Blind.

Kelleher, D. K. (1979, May). Orientation to low vision aids. *Journal of Visual Impairment and Blindness, 73* (5), 161-166.

The Lighthouse Low Vision Service. (1976). *Low Vision Service* (pamphlet). New York: The New York Association for the Blind.

The Lighthouse National Center for Vision and Aging. (1985). *A Better View of You* (pamphlet). Supported by a grant from the Administration on Aging of the U.S. Department of Health and Human Services, New York.

Markle, R. J. (1977). *Household Arts* (professional series 3). Pittsburgh: The Greater Pittsburgh Guild for the Blind.

Slogan, L. L. (1971). *Recommended Aids for the Partially Sighted* (rev. ed.) (Catalogue No. P405). New York: National Society for the Prevention of Blindness, Inc.

Vopata, A. & Wiener, W. (1980, February). Suggested curriculum for distance vision training with optical aids. *Journal of Visual Impairment and Blindness, 74* (2), 49-56.

Wehrum, M. E. (1977). *Techniques of Daily Living* (professional series 5). Pittsburgh: The Greater Pittsburgh Guild for the Blind.

Yeadon, A. & Grayson, D. (1979). *Living with Impaired Vision: An Introduction*. New York: American Foundation for the Blind.

The Certified Occupational Therapy Assistant as an Activity Director

Alice Krawcyk, COTA

SUMMARY. This article will discuss the philosophy and purpose of a Social Adult Day Care Program designed primarily for elderly citizens who may be frail, isolated, or in need of socialization and for their families, who wish to keep elderly relatives at home as long as possible. A second purpose is to maintain the "health" and independence of healthy senior citizens.

The role of the Certified Occupational Therapy Assistant who is the Activity Director of this program will also be explored. The Social Adult Day Care Program is currently offered as a satellite program of the Homemaker Service of Orange County, Inc., in New York, with some funding, support and volunteer assistance provided by a variety of federal, state, and local public and non-profit agencies and voluntary organizations.

This article will discuss the philosophy and structure of a Social Adult Day Care Program (ADC) which has been developed to motivate, encourage, and refer for rehabilitation elderly persons who are impaired as a result of the aging process. It is based on a concept of caring for the elderly who may be frail, isolated, or in need of socialization, and it enables families to keep elderly persons at home for as long as possible. A second goal of the ADC is to maintain the health and independence of "healthy" seniors.

Alice Krawcyk is Activity Director of the Social Adult Day Care Program offered by the Homemaker Service of Orange County, Inc., NY.

The author acknowledges with appreciation the help of Mildred Beard, a volunteer secretary with the Retired Senior Volunteer Program (R.S.V.P.).

This article appears jointly in *Certified Occupational Therapy Assistants: Opportunities and Challenges* (The Haworth Press, 1988) and *Occupational Therapy in Health Care*, Volume 5, Numbers 2/3 (1988).

The article will also discuss the responsibilities and contributions of a Certified Occupational Therapy Assistant (COTA) as the Activity Director of the ADC program. In this particular program the COTA, as Activity Director, is responsible for the structure of the ADC, its social aspects, and related support services and is responsible for program coordination, supervision, assessment, and documentation.

BACKGROUND OF THE SOCIAL ADULT DAY CARE PROGRAM

The Social Adult Day Care Program is a satellite program of the Homemaker Service of Orange County, Inc. (Homemaker Service), a not-for-profit agency. The program was developed as a result of the increasing needs to provide assistance for the elderly and their families.

The elderly have a longer lifespan, which creates needs for assistance, and because of today's high costs of living, it is frequently necessary for both caregivers in a family to work, thereby creating a need for respite care for families. In addition, more families now choose the option of keeping elderly relatives at home for as long as possible because of the increased costs of institutional or nursing home care, which is often limited, or because of their love and concern for them.

As these and other factors were identified as problems in caring for the elderly, options for their care were explored. Health Agency staffs quickly recognized that they could not meet the demands for one-to-one client-staff care in the homes of elderly citizens, but it was found that a supervisor and three assistants could handle up to 20 patients a day in the facilities of the Homemaker Service. Bringing elderly citizens to such a facility could help defray medical costs for both the community and individual families.

Cost savings were important in the establishment of this program, because Medicare does not cover social model ADC programs. The Homemaker Service allocated funds to initiate the program, and donations of equipment, crafts, materials, and money were made by civic groups. Other resources were obtained from the Orange County Office for the Aging (OFA) which provides some grants for low income senior citizens, based on a sliding income scale. OFA also provides some transportation through the Senior Shuttle which operates within the city limits. The Orange County Public Health Department (through Long Term Home Health Care) can provide some reimbursement through Medicaid. The Federal Government can reimburse staff salaries of Title V employees who are over 55 years of age, meet income requirements, and work a maximum of 25 hours. Finally, clients in higher income brackets are charged for participation in the ADC program.

PURPOSE OF THE SOCIAL ADULT DAY CARE PROGRAM

The purpose of the Social Adult Day Care Program is to motivate, encourage, and refer for rehabilitation those elderly who are impaired by the aging process and who may be frail, isolated, or in need of socialization. It also seeks to maintain the health and independence of "healthy" seniors.

The ADC provides care during the daytime in a structured setting away from the adult's home. The program is conducted in a supportive setting in which structured activities are designed to meet the individual needs of its elderly clients. These structured activities not only teach the elderly new skills while they engage in crafts, but they also enable the elderly to relearn activities of daily living and self-care. For many of its clients, the ADC provides a reason for getting up in the morning and enhances their motivation to participate in the day's activities. The ADC program is an approach to maintain and/or increase the independence of elderly persons and provides them with opportunities for socialization.

The clients who participate in the ADC program are often like those elderly citizens who attend programs at a Senior Citizen's Center, except that clients in the ADC program are occasionally handicapped by a physical or mental problem, such as depression, paralysis, or visual and/or hearing disabilities. Clients may need encouragement or re-education to live as normally as possible. A confused client, for example, may need more structure to perform activities, and so a step-by-step procedure may be used to help that client accomplish tasks. Opportunities for successful first ventures may encourage clients to participate in future activities. Along with supervision and structure, clients receive understanding, patience, and empathy from the staff.

ADMISSION OF CLIENTS TO THE ADULT DAY CARE PROGRAM

Eligibility criteria for the Adult Day Care Program state that the client must be socially isolated, able to function in an ambulatory care setting, able to participate in group activities, require some assistance with activities of daily living and in structuring time and activities, and be able to use the bathroom independently.

The Activity Director completes an application which assesses the physical and mental condition of clients who meet the above criteria. This is followed by a personal interview with the applicant responding to questions whenever possible and utilizing the assistance of the caregiver only when necessary. An interest sheet is completed which provides background information about the client and which is used to help plan ADC program activities for the client. Release forms and financial agreements are completed and signed by the responsible person, and an updated physical examination form is required.

While the referring physician can make a verbal order, a written medical history which includes the client's physical condition, diagnoses, list of medications, and physical and dietary restrictions must be completed as soon as possible. The information on this form is checked by the Activity Director and a Registered Nurse, who is a supportive staff member only and who is available for questions when needed. The family must put medications in individual containers, and the Activity Director can remind clients when to take their medications.

A summary of the evaluation and interview is prepared and filed so that activity aides can review the data for background information. A chart is maintained for each client during enrollment in the ADC program, and monthly progress notes document each client's progress. A Discharge Summary report is prepared when the client leaves the program. After one year of program participation, an updated physical report is required, along with an updated assessment and progress notes.

TEAM EFFORT

Members of the ADC team, which consists of a senior activity aide, two activity aides, and volunteers under the supervision of the Activity Director, work together to maintain and increase the mental and physical abilities of clients to prevent or delay institutionalization. Client-centered activities encourage physical and mental participation as well as social interaction.

Open communications are extremely important as they provide both staff and clients an opportunity to deal with relevant concerns, to get feedback, to share ideas, and to work well with one another. Group therapy principles are also vital as staff members must be able to work with clients in a group or to give individual attention when needed.

The staff members plan, organize, and work closely with clients on specific activities, and the staff may supervise a group while a client teaches or demonstrates a craft activity with which the client is familiar. This gives clients opportunities to get involved in the group and to share their life experiences with others in meaningful ways. The staff's ability to utilize socialization skills and interaction help develop rapport within the group.

Staff members and clients, utilizing principles of group therapy and open communications, share ideas and work well together, thereby contributing to client participation in physical, mental and social activities.

THE STRUCTURED DAY

Presently, clients can remain at the facility from 7:30 a.m. until 4:30 p.m., which provides some flexibility for caregivers without interfering with their work schedules. The ADC program operates from 8:00 a.m. until 4:00 p.m.

Days which are scheduled and structured provide orientation for clients as they engage in activities associated with work, play, leisure and self-care. For example, social and group activities centered around arts and crafts, yoga, or discussion of current events provide much needed interaction with peers, which reduces stress and anxiety during other group interactions. However, it is also important for the staff to be flexible and have the ability to make changes if needed.

While there are variations in daily activities, a typical day might begin with a coffee hour and time for socialization to welcome clients as they arrive. Other morning activities might include a discussion of current events, activities designed for reality orientation, body movement, and craft activities. These types of activities are selected because the clients are alert and ready to participate and because they stimulate and enhance growth in communication skills.

Lunch preparations involve client participation, when possible, to provide involvement in meaningful and purposeful tasks. Lunch, itself, is provided through Meals on Wheels, which is a non-profit agency.

Following lunch, the staff provide "Private Time" so that clients can discuss any problems or concerns with staff members or relate happy, exciting events without staff intervention. The day may end with music, card or board games, leisure programs, sitting or walking outside (weather permitting), a discussion group, or with entertainment or a health or educational program. A snack may also be served.

The elderly find camaraderie through socialization with their peers, which enhances their self-esteem and promotes their community involvement. Some of the higher functioning clients volunteer through the Retired Senior Volunteer Program (R.S.V.P.) by participating in small community endeavors such as collating, stuffing, and stamping envelopes. Projects such as these provide excellent opportunities for building self-confidence, self-worth, and restoration of dignity. They also give clients an opportunity to see themselves as valuable citizens and to be recognized as valuable citizens by their community.

REFERRAL SERVICES ASSOCIATED WITH THE ADC PROGRAM

The social ADC program can be a link to referral services for clients and their caregivers. When indicated, clients can be referred to service providers such as physical, occupational, or speech therapists, social workers, adult protective services, or pastoral services.

Caregivers may also be encouraged to participate in support groups such as Alzheimer's groups, Visually Handicapped Social Clubs, and Stroke Clubs.

ROLE OF THE COTA AS ACTIVITY DIRECTOR

The educational background and preparation of Certified Occupational Therapy Assistants uniquely prepares them to serve in the capacity of an Activity Director of programs such as the Adult Day Care Program. It provides knowledge about program development, client referral services, assessing client needs, supervising the activity of staff and aides, and contacting caregivers and physicians. More specifically, educational preparation of COTAs includes interviewing techniques, observational skills, verbal and nonverbal communications, knowledge of medical terminology and the ability to extract appropriate information from medical records and related documents, report writing that is legible, concise, descriptive, and accurate for future references and legal purposes, problem-solving techniques, work simplification techniques, and functional restoration programming.

The minimum qualifications for an Activity Director are completion of an Associate of Arts degree, or its equivalent, knowledge and experience with recreational activities, experience working with the elderly, and certification in cardio-pulmonary resuscitation.

Responsibilities inherent in the Activity Director's position include such things as coordinating, supervising, and directing the Activities Program, coordinating, supervising, and directing aides and volunteers, recruiting both volunteers and clients, maintaining and ordering supplies as well as keeping records of supplies, interviewing prospective clients and coordinating their assessments for eligibility, conducting staff meetings and in-service training, preparing reports, monitoring and recording clients' physical and behavioral changes in progress notes, making recommendations for program development and expansion to the Program Director, contacting caregivers regarding client medication and/or changes in functioning, handling referrals to physicians and other agencies, and submitting regular reports to the ADC Coordinator.

The COTA as Activity Director has important responsibilities in caring for the elderly through programs such as the Adult Day Program described in this article and is uniquely qualified to perform these responsibilities.

CONCLUSION

Because increasing numbers of elderly are remaining with their nuclear families, programs such as the Adult Day Care Program not only contribute to the maintenance of health and independence of the elderly, but they also provide "respite" services for caregivers, who also need support and information concerning the kinds of assistance needed by their elderly relatives or dependents. The Adult Day Care Program has given many elderly the opportunity to remain in their home communities with their own families and has often provided services that would not be available elsewhere.

The Adult Day Care Program described in this paper has worked with clients who have returned to independent lives, using their families as support systems rather than being dependent upon them. Some clients have gone to group homes or have obtained shared housing to live with peers. Some clients have obtained part-time jobs and are now part of the work-force in the community, which enables them to help with their own financial support. Other clients no longer attend the ADC program. These examples are evidence of the growth of clients who have participated in the ADC program. They also provide data to support the growth of Adult Day Care programs as a vital part of care services for the elderly in the future.

A Certified Occupational Therapy Assistant's Contribution to a Substance Abuse Treatment Program

Karen Kunz, COTA

SUMMARY. Substance abuse patients lack skills in money management and frequently misuse credit cards and checks. They also often neglect physical exercise and are in poor physical condition. A COTA developed special programs to teach exercise and money management as part of a five week treatment program for substance abuse patients. Development and implementation of the programs are described.

INTRODUCTION

All members of the Department of Occupational Therapy of the University of Texas Medical Branch are expected to implement a special project in their work settings (Clakeley, 1988; Puccetti, 1988). This article will describe the special projects of the certified occupational therapy assistant in the substance abuse program. A comprehensive treatment program for patients who are substance abusers has many components (Lindsay, 1983). Many substance abusers and psychiatric patients in general are noted to lack physical tolerance (King, 1974), and many patients had asked for help with money problems. Therefore, two components of the substance abuse program were implemented by the assistant for the special project. They were money management and physical exercise programs.

Karen Kunz is assigned to the Substance Abuse Program in the Psychiatry Division of the Department of Occupational Therapy at the University of Texas Medical Branch in Galveston, TX 77550-2777.

This article appears jointly in *Certified Occupational Therapy Assistants: Opportunities and Challenges* (The Haworth Press, 1988) and *Occupational Therapy in Health Care*, Volume 5, Numbers 2/3 (1988).

MONEY MANAGEMENT PROGRAM

Patients with substance abuse problems often have money management problems and need to develop new skills to manage their incomes successfully. If the initial evaluation by the therapist indicates budgeting is a problem for the patient, the patient is referred to the money management program implemented by an assistant.

Program Development and Implementation

The money management program was formulated following many requests from patients for help with money management. In order to learn about finance planning, the assistant made inquiries about community resources. This included visits to banks, and contacting Welfare, housing offices, and food stamp bureaus to learn requirements for their community assistance programs. The local credit bureau was also consulted regarding credit card abuse and hot checks and their legal implications as these problems occur frequently among substance abusers.

The goals of the money management program are to:

1. Increase awareness of the effectiveness of a good money management plan.
2. Improve self-regard by providing successful experiences that involve money, i.e., opening a bank account, grocery shopping, or developing a budget.
3. Decrease anxiety by providing alternatives available for each individual problem.

In the initial evaluation the occupational therapist asks some of the following questions to determine whether or not money management is a problem for the patient. Has the patient ever had checking or savings accounts, and what success did the patient have with them? How well could the patient use household budgets? Who handles the finances in the family and what difficulties have been identified? Does the individual have any concept of a budget or its uses? Is there any understanding of the need to have a plan for using one's money effectively? If there is a problem, the patient is referred to the money management program conducted by the certified occupational therapy assistant.

The initial contact after referral is done on an individual basis. This contact consists of reviewing a personal budget, developing a savings and spending plan, and discussing the patient's ability to pay a bill with a check or a money order. Once the patient demonstrates an understanding of these concepts, a packet of information on money management is provided to the patient. It includes instructions for:

1. calculating personal income;
2. calculating fixed expenses;
3. determination of changing expenses; and
4. setting goals.

The program can be completed in three one hour sessions.

When the patient can plan a monthly budget with this information, he has accomplished the program's goals and is discharged from this treatment segment. Practical experiences are considered for patients who require further assistance.

For example, the grocery store is a major spending area, and a visit to a grocery store near the hospital is used to develop a grocery list. The grocery list is developed to plan food purchases for one month for an individual living alone in preparation for discharge planning. Other practical experiences are planned, such as visits to banks or credit unions to practice opening accounts and dealing with cash.

Another aspect of money management is the difficulty substance abuse patients have in paying for abused credit card charges and hot checks. Patients are encouraged to contact their creditors or community credit counselors if this is a specific problem area for them and they have requested assistance. Often patients are concerned about the legal implications and need reassurance that most creditors will work with an individual and have payment plans available to match the individual's income. Community support groups assist the patient in making contact with agencies that are available in most communities. The patients are given local numbers they can call to set up appointments following discharge.

Results of Money Management Program

Assistance in managing money enables the patient to feel more secure in preparing for discharge and to have the feeling that he will be able to take care of himself with his income.

EXERCISE PROGRAM

Occupational therapists are directly involved in assisting patients to become aware of their physical limitations and to improve physical fitness to carry out physical and emotional daily living skills and to promote a sense of well-being.

The exercise program was developed for substance abuse and general psychiatric populations. The therapist and assistant identified the following problems by clinical observation. There was a noted lack of physical tolerance. Balance was greatly affected through either drug use or physical complications. There was a decrease in the individual's ability to cross midline. There was a lack of motivation generally due to depression. There was an increase in agitation, anxiety secondary to withdrawal and/or cravings. These observations agree with Clark's report (1981) that inactivity resulted in fatigue, physiological inefficiency, poor musculature, inadequate flexibility, and low back pain. And, there was an overall disregard for exercise as being a significant part of a daily routine.

Description of Program

The exercise program has been implemented with a substance abuse unit as well as other psychiatric populations. The assistant is responsible for up to twenty patients from the substance abuse unit. Upon admission to the substance abuse unit a referral is written for occupational therapy to involve the patient in the structured program offered. The exercise program, which begins at 7:15 a.m., is the assistant's first opportunity to meet and observe the patient within the physical fitness group setting. Both specific and general evaluations are done at this time. These include appearance, mood/affect, functional motor, range of motion, mobility, strength and endurance, gross and fine coordination. From these evaluations the following information is documented by the assistant:

General appearance: dress, grooming, hygiene, affect
Range of motion: (active) interferes or does not interfere with performance of daily tasks
Balance: (both sides: amount calculated in seconds)
Endurance: maximum number of repetitions, level of difficulty
Gross motor observations: able or unable to imitate simple movements; able to imitate complex movements, ability to cross midline, patient's gait
Strength and endurance: (in relationship to completing exercise, daily tasks, work, etc.)

The adult exercise program begins with a five minute walk to the exercise facility. The patients sign in to obtain participation points. The program works on a privilege system; they earn one hour passes for their participation with a group. Each individual obtains a mat and is responsible for putting the mat away at the end of the session. The program consists of performing at least eight repetitions, if possible, of each exercise. The assistant leads the patients in a routine program. The following exercises are done:

1. Upper extremity stretches—approximately 10 different ones;
2. Arm exercises (8 with 10 counts each);
3. Waist exercises (6 with 10-20 counts each);
4. Jogging (45-60 seconds);
5. Jumping jacks (15-20);
6. Lower extremity stretches (6 with 10 count);
7. Leg exercises (6 with 10 count);
8. Stomach exercises (4 with 15 count); and
9. Cool down (8 with 8 count).

During these exercises patients are encouraged to count, take deep breaths at suggested intervals and to be aware of any complications they might be having, such as shortness of breath, increased sweating, or dizziness. The patients then return to their unit which includes another five minute walk.

At the request of the therapist, findings are finalized after the assistant has gathered information from actual observation and has interviewed patients briefly on their initial physical or emotional reactions to the exercise program. The patients are also given feedback concerning their performance and offered any suggestions, if necessary. If there are physical concerns dealing with hypertension or seizures, they are referred to the medical staff, and a conclusion is made between the medical staff, assistant and patient. If there are special precautions such as seizure disorders, chronic back pain, physical injury secondary to work or prior altercations, these are also dealt with on an individual basis with the medical staff, assistant and patient.

Goals of the Exercise Program

The following are possible goals of the exercise program for the individuals during treatment:

1. Patient is on time, dressed appropriately and participating in exercise five times weekly.
2. Patient will maximize current range of motion during five week program, if indicated by assessment.
3. Patient will improve balance up to eight seconds – both right and left sides – by two weeks, if indicated.
4. Patient will be able to cross midline and imitate simple movements, as indicated.
5. Patient will be able to complete at least ten repetitions of each exercise for four weeks.

Other goals are also formulated as specific to each patient. Following a two week period the patient's performance is re-evaluated with the same evaluation technique. The patient continues to participate in the exercise program even if goals are dropped from the treatment plan by the therapist as the patient accomplishes these. At time of discharge the patient is interviewed to determine his feelings about his physical condition and about the program itself. A home program is provided if the assistant or the patient indicates this is necessary.

CONCLUSION

Poor money management and lack of exercise resulting in poor physical fitness have been identified as common problems among patients who are substance abusers.

Substance abusers frequently lack the ability to manage money because of impulsive and unwise spending that causes familial and personal problems. A sequence for learning money management by these patients was described. This included teaching modules for budgeting, experiential shopping excursions, and how to obtain referral to community resources for help with money management problems after discharge from the program.

Because inactivity has been linked to various medical and muscular disabilities, an exercise program was added to a comprehensive substance program to prevent these problems. The program content was outlined and patient response described.

REFERENCES

Clakeley, G.L. (1988). Designing job enrichment projects. *Occupational Therapy in Health Care, 5*(2/3), 47-53.

Clark, C. (1981). *Enhancing wellness*. New York: Springer Publishing Company.

King, L.J. (1974). A sensory-integrative approach to schizophrenia. *American Journal of Occupational Therapy, 28*, 529-536.

Lindsay, W.P. (1983). The role of the occupational therapist in the treatment of alcoholism. *American Journal of Occupational Therapy, 37*, 36-43.

Puccetti, D. (1988). Supervision of the certified occupational therapy assistant: developing a knowledge base and strategy. *Occupational Therapy in Health Care, 5*(2/3), 23-35.

Role Delineation of the Registered Occupational Therapist and the Certified Occupational Therapy Assistant in Child Psychiatry

Debora A. Davidson, OTR
Babette C. Lemons, COTA

SUMMARY. This article describes the complementary roles of Registered Occupational Therapists and Certified Occupational Therapy Assistants working in an inpatient child psychiatry unit. Collaborative functions include assessment, treatment, program development and evaluation, and supervision. Supervisory strategies are also described.

INTRODUCTION

Forming and functioning together as members of a working team presents special challenges when team members are of differing educational and experiential backgrounds. This university-affiliated child psychiatry occupational therapy team has developed a team

---

Debora A. Davidson is a team leader, Child and Adolescent Psychiatry Team, Department of Occupational Therapy, University of Texas Medical Branch in Galveston, TX.

Babette C. Lemons was an advanced assistant, Child and Adolescent Psychiatry Team in the Department of Occupational Therapy, University of Texas Medical Branch in Galveston, TX. She is currently a Therapeutic Activities Specialist in the same program.

Appreciation is extended to Lillian Hoyle Parent, MA, OTR, for her encouragement and assistance in writing this paper.

This article appears jointly in *Certified Occupational Therapy Assistants: Opportunities and Challenges* (The Haworth Press, 1988) and *Occupational Therapy in Health Care*, Volume 5, Numbers 2/3 (1988).

model which blends the roles of Registered Occupational Therapists (therapist) and Certified Occupational Therapy Assistants (assistant) so that members' expertise and interests combine to yield sophisticated service delivery. In this paper role delineation will be described in terms of clinical practice, program development, and supervision.

Occupational therapy in inpatient child psychiatry provides opportunities for therapists and assistants to develop a wide range of programming. On a twelve bed unit for children five to thirteen years, a large multidisciplinary team including two therapists and one assistant provides evaluation and treatment of children with problems of social/emotional development, sensorimotor functioning, and daily living skills. The occupational therapy modalities include clinic groups, self-care training, exercise groups, stress management training, and individual and family sessions.

The role delineation between the therapist and assistant is well established and characterized by similarities and differences. The therapist administers and scores standardized evaluations such as the *Bruininks-Oseretsky Test of Motor Proficiency* and the *Piers-Harris Children's Test of Self Concept*; the assistant or therapist administers non-standardized tools such as an interest-skills checklist and task observations. The therapist and assistant collaborate in developing a list of assets and problems. The therapist formulates and writes the evaluation report and treatment plan with input from the assistant and is responsible for sharing these in clinical team meetings.

The assistant's responsibilities are almost entirely clinical, with few of the administrative or teaching tasks that the therapist's role includes. The assistant works daily with all of the children and thus is a consistent source of information about patients' progress. Additionally, because the assistant conducts a morning Daily Living Skills program on the ward, she has frequent interaction with nursing and child care staff. This link with another part of the multidisciplinary team is most informative and helpful in identifying and preventing minor administrative and clinical conflicts. The therapist establishes a more formal link to the multidisciplinary team via participation in administrative and planning meetings.

SPECIALIZED PROGRAM DEVELOPMENT

The morning Daily Living Skills Program was initiated after various clinical team members expressed concerns about the children's grooming, appearance and mealtime behaviors. The therapist and assistant met with nursing staff to identify specific needs and to discuss logistical issues such as schedules and staffing patterns. The assistant then designed a program proposal which included (1) goals (to increase children's independence in grooming and dressing and to improve mealtime manners, which would impact social functioning and self-concept) and (2) methods (skill training, monitoring and motivating via a behavioral charting and reward system). An evaluation form, which allowed for qualitative assessment of daily living skills and denoted normative age ranges for skills acquisition, was developed for pre- and post-testing (see Figure 1). The proposal was presented by the therapist to the head nurse and then to the entire multidisciplinary administrative staff prior to its implementation. Feedback from nursing and child care staff was sought by the assistant and the therapist throughout the first stage of program implementation.

The benefits of this program have been many. Formal evaluation revealed that one-third to one-half of the patient groups have poorly developed self-care and mealtime skills and can benefit from the training program. Children have developed significantly improved self-concepts, as indicated by positive remarks about their appearance, and have become more popular with adults and peers at mealtime due to improved table manners. In addition, the collaborative working relationship between occupational therapy and nursing has been enhanced.

Part of this program has been developed into a Quality Assurance study. The therapists and assistant have developed a form which details observable components of appropriate table manners, and have established inter-rater reliability. The occupational therapy staff are sharing data-gathering responsibilities, and the therapist organizes and analyzes the data for occupational therapy team review and interpretation. Results are compiled for presentation at the Occupational Therapy Department's monthly Quality Assurance Meeting and may serve as a pilot for a larger study.

DATE: ____________

NAME: ____________

AGE: ____________

DRESSING	RATING SCALE	Independent	Verbal Cue Required	Needs Assistance	Dependent	Neat	Messy	Comments
1. Clean clothes	(10.0)							
2. Clean socks	(10.0)							
3. Matched clothes	(8.6–9.0)							
4. Belt in loops	(7.0)							
5. Shoes tied	(7.0)							
6. Shirt or dress buttoned	(3.6)							
7. Clothing fastened	(4.0)							
8. Wearing undergarments								
GROOMING								
1. Washes face	(5.0–6.0)							
2. Brushes teeth	(4.0–5.0)							
3. Combs hair	(5.0–6.0)							
4. Uses deodorant	(9.6–10.0)							
5. Cleans nose	(5.0)							
6. Washes hands	(8.0)							
EATING								
1. Uses spoon								
2. Uses fork	(5.6–6.0)							
3. Cleans table afterwards	(4.6)							
4. Uses napkins	(6.6–7.0)							
5. Eats with mouth closed	(10.0)							
6. Uses knife	(7.6–8.0)							
7. Stays seated	(9.0)							

FIGURE 1. Child Psychiatry ADL Checklist

Developmental norms (Rating Scale Above) taken from: Cohen, M. and Gross, P.: *The Developmental Resource: Behavioral Sequences & Program Planning*, Vol. II, Grune & Stratton, New York, 1975.

SUPERVISION

In this setting supervision occurs in several ways. There are formal meetings between the supervising therapist and the assistant at least twice per month, during which the assistant's special projects, continuing education interests and clinical skills are discussed. Team clinical meetings are held weekly to review treatment and program planning. Finally, functioning as co-therapists in groups every day establishes a working relationship based on observation and appreciation of each team member's role and the effective delineation of functions among the members of the OTR-COTA Team.

CONCLUSION

This paper illustrates how therapists and assistants have worked together to develop and deliver clinically sophisticated programming. Developing a team which is structured to have adequate role overlap to allow continuity of care, while simultaneously promoting expression of individual interests and skills presents a challenge which is rewarded by clinical superiority and worker satisfaction.

The Roles of the Certified Occupational Therapy Assistant and the Registered Occupational Therapist in Adult Psychiatry

Christine Johnson, OTR
Catherine Santos, COTA

SUMMARY. The certified occupational therapy assistant in a 64 bed inpatient psychiatry setting contributes to a high level of patient care and departmental efficiency. The certified occupational therapy assistant's responsibilities include direct patient care, student education, and clinical management and are described in this article. The methods and philosophy for supervision of the certified occupational therapy assistant are explored. In conclusion, two adult psychiatry programs which utilize the Certified Occupational Therapy Assistant's knowledge and education are described.

INTRODUCTION

The importance of certified occupational therapy assistants (assistants) to the practice of occupational therapy in adult psychiatry is immeasurable. The assistants ensure that occupational therapy

---

Christine Johnson is Supervisor of Adult Inpatient Psychiatry in The Department of Occupational Therapy at the University of Texas Medical Branch, Galveston, TX 77550-2777.

Catherine Santos previously was Assistant in Adult Inpatient Psychiatry. She is now Assistant in the Adult Outpatient Psychiatry Program in the Department of Occupational Therapy at the University of Texas Medical Branch, Galveston, TX 77550-2777.

This article appears jointly in *Certified Occupational Therapy Assistants: Opportunities and Challenges* (The Haworth Press, 1988) and *Occupational Therapy in Health Care*, Volume 5, Numbers 2/3 (1988).

treatment plans are implemented accurately, that students and aides receive feedback about their daily performance, and that the occupational therapy clinical area is operated in a systematic and effective manner.

The adult psychiatry program at the University of Texas Medical Branch (UTMB) receives referrals from a 64 bed hospital with six adult psychiatric inpatient units: the intensive care unit; acute care unit, general psychiatric unit, older adult unit, substance abuse unit, and clinical research unit. There are four assistant (COTA) and seven registered occupational therapist (OTR) positions providing services for adult psychiatric care in the Occupational Therapy Department.

STAFF RESPONSIBILITIES

Each professional working in this large occupational therapy department has responsibilities to ensure that optimal, safe, and effective patient care is provided. Many of these responsibilities are shared and some are assigned to specific persons. The therapists and assistants work cooperatively to develop new and innovative treatment programs and groups as the needs arise within the patient population.

Therapist Responsibilities

The therapist's role in this program is to conduct the initial evaluations and develop treatment plans and goals based on results and conclusions drawn from the evaluations. The treatment program is then implemented to achieve these goals. The therapist will provide individual treatment for those patients who are in her caseload or may delegate some of these responsibilities to an assistant.

The therapist's responsibilities include the supervision of Level I and Level II fieldwork students and inservices to medical and nursing students, staff and residents concerning the importance of occupational therapy in the center setting.

Assistant Responsibilities

The responsibilities of the assistant in this setting are varied and rewarding. Assistants are involved in direct patient care from the time of the patient's initial referral to occupational therapy through the patient's discharge. Assistants also help the therapists initiate and conduct the initial evaluations and provide basic evaluative information to the occupational therapist who will establish the initial plan and goals for the patient.

After the therapist establishes the treatment plan, the assistant implements a treatment program and follows through with the goals established as a result of the initial evaluation. The assistant may provide individual treatment to those patients assigned to her in areas such as budgeting, self-care activities, job preparation skills, and safety issues (as indicated in the original initial evaluation goals).

The assistants lead or co-lead the treatment groups provided by occupational therapy. The assistants can lead the craft groups, communication groups, exercise groups, and self-care groups. The assistant acquires knowledge about the various treatment approaches to group therapy in the following ways: attending continuing education courses on a specific topic, reading a variety of professional journals and books on the specific topic, and by attending the group itself and observing other occupational therapy personnel lead the group. The groups may be run by two assistants (at least one with experience in that group) or by an assistant and a therapist.

The experienced assistant may perform evaluations of the patient's cooking abilities, self-care skills or safety precaution awareness without the immediate direct supervision of a therapist. In addition to direct patient care, assistants with experience are assigned additional responsibilities, such as: providing supervision of OT and COTA students, student workers, and aides; maintaining the budget for each clinical area, and ordering adequate materials and supplies for effective patient care.

Shared Responsibilities

Interdisciplinary team rounds are attended alternately by the assistant and the therapist to provide feedback to the team members concerning the patients' performances. The assistant's role in communicating information from the interdisciplinary team members to the occupational therapy team is essential to ensure effective and efficient patient care.

In many instances the responsibilities of the assistant and the therapist overlap and complement each other. Effective patient care is the ultimate outcome of close collaboration between the therapist and the assistant.

SUPERVISION

Supervision is provided in many forms and includes written performance appraisals, weekly team meeting, weekly individual supervisory sessions, and intermittent informal feedback. Each supervisory session emphasizes active participation by the assistant and the supervisor. Either the assistant or the supervisor may bring up issues, plans or concerns to be discussed. Participatory supervision is emphasized so that each participant assumes responsibility in the decision making process.

Written Performance Appraisal

The written performance appraisal is completed annually. This evaluation focuses on those professional behaviors and responsibilities that the Occupational Therapy Department staff have determined are an integral part of the assistant's job description. The assistant brings to this supervisory session ideas for professional growth and personal goals for the upcoming year.

Weekly Team Meetings

Occupational therapists and assistants working in specified areas hold weekly team meetings. These meetings fulfill a variety of purposes. Information can be passed from the supervisor to the other team members, issues between staff members can be discussed, program development can occur, and productive staff development is ensured through sharing new information.

Individual Supervisory Sessions

Individual supervisory sessions are also conducted on a weekly basis. The emphasis of these meetings is to promote development of the assistant's personal goals developed for the year. The assistant and the supervisor work together to develop and implement the assistant's plan of action for reaching specified goals. Any positive or constructive feedback concerning the assistant's performance of professional duties within the last week is provided at this time. The assistant also gives feedback to the supervisor about the supervision received.

In a large department such as the one at UTMB, all assistants and therapists give and receive feedback from their peers. As an assistant becomes more familiar with the treatment setting and its routines, less direct supervision is necessary, and both the therapist and the assistant work together harmoniously. It is not always possible for the casual observer to identify a distinct difference between what the therapist and the assistant each do. This is especially true of a team where rapport between the two enables them to work together without obvious differentiation of roles. Differentiation always exists in the program and follows the American Occupational Therapy Association's role delineation guidelines (AOTA, 1981) and state licensing requirements (Vernon, 1984).

PROGRAM EXAMPLES

Program for Older Adult Patients in Psychiatry

This facility offers a variety of programs. Two of the programs will be described. The first will be the Older Adult program. This is a program for psychiatric patients over fifty-five years of age. These patients may have a variety of mental and physical diagnoses and levels of cognitive abilities. The treatment program includes physical activities to facilitate kinesthetic, vestibular, and proprioceptive responses. Adult games promote active listening, cooperation among group members, and cognitive functioning. Cooking sessions provide sensory stimulation and encourage each patient to continue involvement in as many daily physical activities as is reasonable.

One of several therapists and the assistant co-lead the group activity. Prior to each session, the therapist and assistant confer to establish each of their roles for that particular session. Following each session the therapists and assistant discuss the session. This may include recording observations of patient behavior, identifying successes or difficulties within the group, and determining whether patient goals which were set by therapist were met.

Self-Care Program for Older Adults in Psychiatry

The second is the self-care program. This program was designed primarily for older adult patients; however, disorganized younger patients are sometimes included in the self-care program. Levels of independence vary from patient to patient. The treatment program includes activities such as bathing and/or showering, washing clothes, washing and/or styling hair, dressing, brushing teeth or dentures, and application of appropriate make-up. The primary goal is to improve each patient's level of independence in performing self-care skills.

The therapist and assistant co-lead the group on a rotating basis. The initial goal is to assess the patients' level of functioning. Verbal or physical assistance is provided to the patient as necessary, and adaptive equipment is provided to enhance a patient's performance. Individual patient performance is discussed with nursing staff to encourage maintenance of acquired levels of performance over the weekends. The final step usually includes discussing the patient's progress with significant others if the patient is to return home. All in all, the most important factor in the self-care program is communicating with other staff on a daily basis about the patient's status since patients are treated by different therapists daily.

CONCLUSION

A small portion of an inpatient psychiatric program has been described. The certified occupational therapy assistants perform important responsibilities. Nevertheless, the roles of the assistant and therapists in this setting complement and support one another. The assistant contributes to provision of optimal patient care, effective student education, and efficient management of the occupational therapy clinical setting. Continuous open communication between the therapists and shared respect for each other make possible these high levels of patient care and department efficiency.

REFERENCES

American Occupational Therapy Association (1981). *Entry level role delineation for OTRs and COTAs*. (Reference Manual of Official Documents of the American Occupational Therapy Association, Inc., VII.1-VII.10). Rockville, MD: American Occupational Therapy Association.

Vernon's Texas Civil Statutes, Article 8851 (1984). Title 40, Texas Administrative Code, Amendment 383.1, d,e,f,g,k. St. Paul, MN: West Publishing Company.

Incorporating Structured Learning Therapy into Occupational Therapy Treatment of Chronic Psychiatric Patients

Wendy Ellen Wallach, COTA
Daniel Hopper, MA

SUMMARY. Role playing activities, when incorporated into a group experience, have been shown to enhance social skills development in patients with chronic psychiatric conditions. This approach, adapted from the psychological therapeutic model of Structured Learning Therapy, addresses interpersonal skill development at three distinct levels: rudimentary interpersonal skills, community interpersonal skills, and abstract interpersonal skills. Unique to this therapeutic model is the concept of the patient taking an active role in formulating the dialogues used in each role playing situation.

In *Skill Training for Community Living: Applying Structured Learning Therapy* (Goldstein, Gershaw & Sprafkin, 1976), the concepts and format for a therapeutic approach designed to teach personal and interpersonal coping and mastery skills are set forth. This therapeutic approach was found to be successful in both inpatient

---

Wendy Ellen Wallach is a member of the American Occupational Therapy Association, the New York State Occupational Therapy Association, and the Rockland County Disability Advisory Council, of which she is secretary. She is currently employed at Rockland Psychiatric Center, Unit for Supportive Rehabilitation, Orangeburg, NY.

Daniel Hopper is a member of the American Psychological Association and Coalition of Hospital and Institutional Psychologists. He is currently employed at Rockland Psychiatric Center, Unit for Supportive Rehabilitation, Orangeburg, NY.

This article appears jointly in *Certified Occupational Therapy Assistants: Opportunities and Challenges* (The Haworth Press, 1988) and *Occupational Therapy in Health Care*, Volume 5, Numbers 2/3 (1988).

and outpatient settings, with the emphasis on assisting persons to lead more satisfying and productive lives through use of improved communication skills. Goldstein, et al., (1976) begin with such basic interpersonal skills as "Starting a Conversation" and gradually moves toward more complex themes such as "Social, Financial, and Personal Aspects of Daily Living." These authors incorporated four basic behavior change components into their therapeutic approach: modeling, role playing, social reinforcement, and transfer training.

The basic format for Structured Learning Therapy (SLT) calls for a group of 8-12 patients to meet from 2-3 times per week for no more than two hours for each session. This approach calls for prerecorded tapes delineating the various steps found to be necessary in dealing with everyday problems to be played at the beginning of each session (the modeling component). The patients are next encouraged to rehearse these dialogues in detail within the group setting in pairs until mastered (the role playing component). Their mastery is further assisted by group discussion of the performance (social reinforcement) and is finally solidified behaviorally by using the newly learned coping or mastery skill in a real life setting (the transfer training component).

Therapy sessions are led by two trainers who alternately instruct and observe the patients through the training phases. Optimal setting for sessions is a room with a neutral environment with patients seated in a half circle around a chalkboard. The trainers take turns observing the role playing, with one trainer seated within the half circle. The other trainer guides the patients through each sequence while standing by the blackboard, on which has been written the steps required for each topic of conversation. At the end of the session, the topics of discussion are to be summarized, and each patient is given a "homework" assignment by the trainers. These assignments are to be reviewed at the beginning of the next session.

The authors continually stress the flexibility of this approach so that it can be applied in a variety of settings and modified to meet specific treatment needs so long as the essential format and structure are maintained.

This therapeutic model was adapted by the authors to respond to the gross deficiencies commonly seen in chronic psychiatric patients who are often unable to carry on meaningful and focused conversations with others.

This type of treatment model is ideal as a tool for use in Occupational Therapy. It is further an excellent activity for a COTA to conduct with another team member as co-trainer. This model successfully incorporates many occupational therapy principles and training techniques that are within the scope of practice for a COTA. Its primary concern is in social skills training, and it is centered around an activity (role playing). Furthermore, abstract social skills are broken down into smaller, specific concrete subskills, which are more easily understood and replicated. In addition, peripheral skills such as listening, problem solving, and reading comprehension are inherent in each exercise undertaken during each phase of the SLT process.

At the onset, patients involved in our training groups were oriented with a pre-discharge frame of reference. Therefore, many of the skills they requested to work on dealt with situations likely to be encountered in the community.

APPLICATION

In applying the method in a rehabilitation unit of a state run inpatient psychiatric facility, eight patients (four males and four females) were selected. Their daily levels of functioning were considered high by both ward staff and physicians, and they were being considered for discharge placement within the following six months. These patients also possessed particular strengths and weaknesses that were felt would add to the group process both in a supportive way and in enabling the trainers to draw upon a variety of training techniques to address those special problems.

The treatment area selected was an unused activity room in the basement of a building adjoining the main clinical area. The room itself was large and well equipped with various types of furniture, blackboards, sinks, and bathrooms. The standard arrangement of chairs and blackboard was used, with the trainers alternating between directing the dialogues with pairs of patients and sitting within the half circle observing from that perspective. Typically sessions lasted ninety minutes, with the last ten minutes devoted to summary discussion of the skills just role played, during which time light refreshments were served.

In our application of the Goldstein et al. method, each interpersonal phase is tailored to meet the specific needs of the patients in the group, although the first training dialogue was the same one used by Goldstein et al. and is entitled "Starting a Conversation." This is a basic skill but was chosen because it clearly defines the procedural aspects of the therapy and is also non-threatening for an initial group activity. There are five basic steps to this concept:

1. choosing the right time and place;
2. greeting the person;
3. making small talk;
4. assessing whether the person is listening and interested; and
5. getting to the main topic.

These steps are written on the blackboard so that the members of the group may refer to them throughout the session.

One trainer explains the purpose of learning the steps for each specific skill and the proceeds to discuss each step listed on the blackboard. When the patients are familiar with the method, the trainers then role play this first dialogue themselves. Next, a pair of patients is selected or volunteers to try the role playing by going through the steps that are listed. When they are finished, the group discusses how well they followed the outline, makes suggestions about what could have been done better, or targets any steps that were omitted. Another pair of patients is then chosen, and the process is repeated until every patient has had a turn at each role that is to be played during that session.

It should be noted that initial hesitations to role play are accepted, and such patients are allowed to wait for another turn. It is made clear, however, that each patient must participate at some point in the session. Only on rare occasions was it necessary for the trainers to employ other techniques, such as arranging for group support or peer pressure to ensure participation.

When each concept had been thoroughly practiced and discussed, the patients were encouraged to practice these newly learned skills in real life settings (i.e., on the ward, in the activities center, on pass). With this method only one or two skills could be introduced during each session. This depended on levels of complexity and whether topics chosen were related to each other.

The therapists noted that after only two or three sessions the group formed a supportive and cohesive union. Patients were more intimate and relaxed with each other. They became the primary advocates for the group and the therapy method. In essence, it appears that as a result of their participation in this group, they felt unique and motivated. They began to tell other patients, both within and out of the rehabilitation unit, about "their" therapy group. As word spread, the trainers were approached by a variety of patients requesting that they, too, be allowed to join the group. Names of these patients were accepted by the trainers as candidates for future groups.

This motivation on the part of the members translated well into the therapy sessions, where the patients began to play a more active role. Initially the trainers presented the first few topics to be discussed. After the third session, the patients were asked if they had any problems in their social communications that they would like to address. A list of ideas was drawn up. From it, the most recurrent problems were extracted as subjects for future sessions. It was left to the patients to formulate the steps for each of these new subjects, a task they were now able to accomplish with a minimum of assistance from the trainers. Such a process not only aided them both in learning and internalizing the step method but also increased their perception that the group belonged to them. It also represented an important step forward in their treatment and eventual discharge.

The use of this method as it applies to each of the three training levels will now be discussed.

INTERPERSONAL SKILLS

The first level, called interpersonal skills, involves itself with the training in basic social skills and with situations focused on encounters with others. It is in this phase that the patient becomes familiar with the SLT process and begins to grasp the idea of how to break communication skills into steps.

Four situations were used in this phase: starting a conversation, talking to your doctor (or other professional), how to meet people at a party or social gathering, and how to deal with flirtations that are directed at your boyfriend/girlfriend. Of these four situations, the first two were proposed by the trainers, with the latter two being proposed by the patients.

At the end of each session, the patients were asked to use the process in their daily interactions. They were encouraged to report their success or failure in the following session. The "homework" experience (or transfer training) used at the end of this phase was a monthly ward party, given by volunteers from a local organization. With both trainers present, each patient was asked to solicit information (such as name, job, family information) from one of the volunteers. Such an experience served to demonstrate, both to the trainers and the patients, competency gained in the phase being completed.

COMMUNITY INTERPERSONAL SKILLS

The second level is titled Community Interpersonal Skills. It is directed to particularly difficult or stressful situations that patients might encounter in the community. At this point in the therapy, members are considered to have become familiar with the step-by-step process so the trainers no longer need to write the steps on the blackboard. Three basic situations were used in this phase: dealing with line jumpers, dealing with difficult waitresses, and dealing with uncooperative salesclerks.

Discussions precede each dialogue dealing with the issue of assertiveness vs. aggressiveness. The "fieldwork" at the end of this phase involves a trip by the group into the community. Accompanied by the trainers, patients are asked to go into various stores and inquire about unpriced items and store policies on such things as returns and hours of operation. In addition, patients are taken to a restaurant for a meal and encouraged to ask a number of specific questions regarding items on the menu. In the first group, this, in fact, did elicit some impatience from the waitress and therefore provided an excellent illustration of how useful their new skills were going to be to them.

ABSTRACT INTERPERSONAL SKILLS

The last level, in which abstract interpersonal skills are the focus, involves patients primarily with those encounters in their daily lives perceived as most difficult and stressful. At this stage, the breakdown of the steps used in the various situations is done by the patients themselves, with the trainer's role being that of guides. Situations used in this level were dealing with another person's loss (death), taking responsibility when another person says he intends to harm himself or another person, what to do when you become the focus of someone else's hallucinations, what to do if someone steals something from you, how to deal with difficult staff members, and how to interview for discharge placement. The content for these topics included such concepts as responsibility for others, delusions and hallucinations, and appropriate channels for voicing complaints.

The conclusion of this three level program was a party for the group. The intent was to leave each of the members with positive memories of the group experience and to reward each member for completing the program. Certifications of merit were awarded at this time and proclaimed that each member had successfully completed the therapy.

DISCUSSION

Structured Learning Therapy, while similar to many other psychological models, has a definite place in Occupational Therapy programming, with the certified occupational therapy assistant being one of the co-trainers and the occupational therapist or psychologist being the second co-trainer. The occupational therapist can also be a mentor, providing supervision when needed.

From an interdisciplinary treatment perspective, both the COTA and psychologist described herein play very distinct roles. Since frequently patients role play real situations, intense feelings and emotion are often evident. It is in this capacity that the psychologist is most useful. He utilizes clinical judgment to determine how these emotional displays should be dealt with and how best to use the dynamics of the group. The COTA's perspective is most important in the step-by-step process of the various interactions, as well as in observing and evaluating transference of skills learned during the various activities in which patients engage.

The key word in the selection of SLT as a treatment modality is its adaptability. It is a process which allows the patients to identify their own problems as subjects for role playing and to formulate their own dialogues based on situations they have previously experienced. This use of the method described in this paper differs from the method used by Goldstein et al., who used preconstructed interactions.

CONCLUSION

In our experience, it is evident that a majority of the chronic psychiatric patients that completed our application of Structured Learning Therapy are able to internalize and transfer skills learned into real life situations. This observation is based on reports from team members and behaviors displayed during transfer training experiences. Patients were able, in most instances, to successfully interact with others in a socially acceptable manner when applying the methods learned. Three groups have completed the program described in this paper, and similar results have been found in each group.

It is strongly recommended that others who apply the method described in this paper should focus on the interpersonal deficits that are most critical for the specific group of patients engaged in the treatment program. These deficits can be adapted to fit the phases outlined and can be worked on with the step-by-step process within the framework of role playing.

REFERENCE

Goldstein, A.P., Gershaw, J.N., and Sprafkin, R.P. (1976). *Skill training for community living: Applying structured learning therapy*. NY: Pergamon.

Job Search Skills for Unemployed Psychiatric Patients

Kathryn E. Wassink, COTA

SUMMARY. Chronically mentally ill patients often lack skills for finding employment independently. A program based on "SCORE: Solving Community Obstacles and Restoring Employment" was implemented by a Certified Occupational Therapy Assistant in a teaching hospital. The program implemented two years ago as a Special Project has been successful. Fifteen low level patients trained in this program have obtained remunerative employment and two others are performing volunteer services on a regular basis.

INTRODUCTION

Historically occupational therapists have planned treatment programs for patients to achieve a balance of work and leisure in their daily lives. Work is often equated with gainful employment, and this goal has been difficult for many mentally ill patients to achieve, especially during times of regional or national unemployment.

Chronic mentally ill patients in remission, who may be out of touch with the mainstream of techniques or procedures for finding and obtaining a job, are particularly vulnerable to the problems of unemployment. Occupational therapists have used various methods to achieve the goal of returning mentally ill patients to work. This paper describes a program conducted by a Certified Occupational

---

Kathryn E. Wassink is employed in the Psychiatry Division of the Occupational Therapy Department of the University of Texas Medical Branch Hospitals, Galveston, TX 77550-2777.

This article appears jointly in *Certified Occupational Therapy Assistants: Opportunities and Challenges* (The Haworth Press, 1988) and *Occupational Therapy in Health Care*, Volume 5, Numbers 2/3 (1988).

Therapy Assistant to teach chronic mentally ill patients to gain independence in obtaining a job.

BACKGROUND

Because chronic mentally ill patients may have lost contact with job-search networks (Watts, 1976), staffs of occupational therapy programs have identified potential placements and then selected patients to work in transitional employment settings (DeMars, 1975). Occupational therapists have also developed contracts for training opportunities for patients (Howe, 1981). While helpful in placing patients in work or training programs, these methods do not make the patient independent or teach job-seeking skills. Teaching patients how to seek employment and to make application or appointments for job interviews is a methodology to make them more independent in the process of obtaining employment.

A report from one occupational therapy program in which patients were taught how to seek employment indicated that the patients achieved only minimal success. The authors suggested that the patients may have had concerns about their abilities to maintain their recovery stage when confronted with the stress and responsibilities of full-time employment. There was perhaps too much psychological risk-taking for the patients (Deacon, Dunning & Dease, 1974). Another problem of mentally ill persons in remission that is associated with seeking jobs and job interviews is a lack of appropriate social behavior and verbal skills to conduct a job interview or inability to answer questions appropriately without saying too much or too little (Watts, 1976).

Occupational therapists have also assessed work potential and work behavior of the mentally ill (Andersen, 1985). Stauffer (1986), among others, has described studies related to evaluation and training programs for this population. Most authors agree that additional investigation is necessary regarding the outcome of occupational therapy treatment associated with work-related training and the outcome results about work potential of the chronic mentally ill. However, general success should be related to the outcome of obtaining and holding a job successfully.

Kramer and Biedel (1982) reported the results of a 10-week job training program designed to teach job seeking skills to a chronic psychiatric population. A year after the program was implemented 16 of 41 subjects were working either for monetary compensation in a job training program or were performing volunteer services. Eighteen of the unemployed were still in active treatment for their mental illness. Kramer (1984) described this program at length in "SCORE: Solving Community Obstacles and Restoring Employment."

WORK PROGRAM: DEVELOPMENT AND IMPLEMENTATION

A Certified Occupational Therapy Assistant II (assistant) in the adult psychiatry program identified needs for a transitional program for chronic psychiatric in-patients as they progressed to out-patient clinics and potential employment. Consequently, she developed a program in early 1985 based on "SCORE: Solving Community Obstacles and Restoring Employment," (hereinafter referred to as SCORE). The content of the program was selected after reviewing literature on occupational therapy and vocational placements of the chronically mentally ill. The SCORE Program (Kramer, 1984) was well outlined and demonstrated some success with a population of chronic psychiatric patients (Kramer & Biedel, 1982).

The program was presented to the total occupational therapy staff in psychiatry. The staff accepted the proposal, and the assistant elected to implement this program for her special project in the fall of 1985. Every staff member selects a special project to contribute to departmental programming (Clakeley, 1988; Puccetti, 1988). The assistant implemented the program with the supervision of the therapist in charge of the occupational therapy program for adult psychiatric patients.

Patients can be referred to the job-search program by a physician or by the occupational therapy staff in any of the occupational therapy units, such as the substance abuse unit, the adult in-patient unit, or the out-patient psychiatric unit. Patients may continue with regular psychiatric and occupational therapy treatment while participating in the job-search program.

Criteria for referral and acceptance into the Job-Search program are that the patient be motivated to seek employment, has demonstrated difficulty locating and maintaining employment, has functional verbal skills, and may be willing to participate in videotaping of role-play sessions. These videotaped role-play sessions are used to help patients identify inappropriate interview behavior. Patients are not excluded for refusing to participate in videotaping but are expected to participate in role-playing interview experiences used to help the patient identify inappropriate interview behavior. However, the patient is expected to participate in role-playing interview experiences.

After referral and placement in a group of two to ten persons, patient groups spend from thirty minutes to two hours one to four times a week working on job-search skills. Some of the preparatory work may be done prior to a patient's discharge, and the patient may complete the program while continuing in the transitional outpatient clinic. The goals for a patient in the job preparation program are to practice and learn the steps necessary to obtain employment and become independent in the use of appropriate skills for each step.

The steps in the job preparation program include preparing a resume, learning where to look for a job and how to fill out application forms, learning to write a letter of application, and obtaining a job interview independently. The job interview is crucial to obtaining employment, and interviewing is a skill which many chronic psychiatric patients may never have acquired or have lost. This program places much emphasis on how the patient communicates the appropriate information that is a crucial part of the job-search process.

The patients in the program are also given extensive skills training, including training for appropriate grooming for the interview and work situation. They learn methods to engage in appropriate conversation for the job interview, the rules of etiquette, and how to accept constructive criticism in conversations. They are taught to be aware of verbal and nonverbal communication.

Tasks associated with each step of the process leading to employment are learned as the patient goes through a series of modules suggested in SCORE (Kramer, 1984). The modules can be completed independently by the patient or with the guidance of the assistant. One or more modules can be worked on concurrently, such as grooming, hygiene and social skills training. Each module and its general tasks are described below.

Data Collection and Evaluation for a Resume

The initial step in obtaining information is to have the patient complete a form to obtain demographic, educational, occupational and leisure information about the patient's background and history. This provides the basic information to be used as a guide to the kind of job or jobs that the patient's work and leisure background indicates may be performed successfully. The patient uses the information from the data collection module to develop a resume. The assistant guides the patient in the writing of the resume. This information leads the patient to the next module.

Job Sources

The second module suggests places where the patient can begin to look for work. This involves discussions about work the patient has ever done or is interested in doing. It is the assistant's responsibility to help the patient narrow the job sought to one specific employment or skill area such as clerk, laborer, or secretary, based on skills the patient may have had prior to illness. After selecting a specific job category, the patient is guided to look through want ads, the telephone book for employment agencies, or for notices of available jobs that might appear outside plants and places of business.

Application Forms

The third module contains a series of application forms, and the patient practices completing those that are most like jobs found in the want ads. Completing the forms requires the patient to identify and collect the essential information needed to complete an application form. Information to be collected includes the patient's social security number, birth certificate, drivers license and, if applicable, military records and education or training certificates. The patient is also instructed to obtain permission from persons he wishes to use as references. A list of words commonly used to complete applications is included in the module to guide the patient in completing the forms. For example, when asked "Who referred you to this job?", the answer is the name of a person who made the referral or "Myself" if the patient is initiating the contact. In the place on the form asking "Date Available," the reply is "Immediately." The response to "Salary Requirement" is "Flexible." "Reasons for leaving previous employment" are listed. The patient is instructed to state whether a specific position is desired, such as mechanic, clerk, dishwasher, or general laborer. Finally, the patient is instructed to write legibly using black ink, to provide all information requested, and to be as truthful and accurate as possible when providing answers to questions.

The assistant reviews the completed application forms and makes suggestions regarding wording and answers to information requested until the patient completes the forms to fulfill criteria for accuracy, legibility and completeness.

Application Letter

In this module the patient concentrates on writing a letter of application according to a designated format. For example, the letter is to be based on a want ad in a local paper. The completed letter is reviewed by the assistant who may suggest changes in format, information, spelling, and correction of grammatical errors.

Interview

After the patient learns to successfully complete the previous steps in the job-search process, this module prepares the patient for an interview. During other treatment times the patient has been instructed in daily hygiene and grooming in order to prepare for the interview. The men were instructed to be clean shaven, and the women were coached in make-up and hair grooming. All were instructed in appropriate dress and cleanliness for the approaching interview. Good self-care is a usual part of the habit training undertaken in the various psychiatric programs in the department. The patients accept this because no one individual is singled out for comment. The importance of cleanliness and good hygiene are emphasized in looking for work.

Watts (1976), describing employment handicaps of the mentally ill, suggested that social behavior and the ability to answer questions appropriately are important assets in obtaining employment. Watts suggested that videotaped interviews might be a way to help patients learn how to conduct themselves in job interviews. The SCORE program (Kramer & Biedel, 1982) describes videotaped role-playing interview sessions, and at the University of Texas Medical Branch (hereinafter referred to as UTMB) videotaping is used in such sessions. The patient is given a series of questions that are often asked during an interview such as "What was your last employment?," "What did you do?," or "What machinery do you operate?"

Upon agreeing to be videotaped, the patient must call the assistant, ask for an interview, and make an appointment. During the scheduled interview, which is videotaped, the assistant plays the role of a personnel officer and the patient is the applicant. A thorough job interview, based on the type of job for which the patient is applying, is conducted. After the interview the videotape is replayed, and the patient is asked to view his performance. The assistant indicates to the patient appropriate or inappropriate behavior during the interview. If additional sessions are necessary, other role-playing interviews are videotaped, and the patient is asked to watch and comment on his own performance based on the guidelines for job interviews. As the patient becomes more able to identify and later correct ineffective behaviors, movements, tics, or inappropriate answers, he moves closer to an actual job-search and interview.

Although most of the behaviors identified above are taken for granted by people in the general population, the psychiatric patient in remission or recovery may have had neither the knowledge nor the experience of using these behaviors. Therefore, it is necessary to rehearse and coach the patient in their use until they become easier and perhaps more habitual behaviors used by the patient.

CASE DESCRIPTION 1

A 32-year-old single male with chronic depression, retrolental fibroplasia and cerebral palsy was admitted to the job-search program. He was hospitalized four years previously and had not held a job for six years. His education included an Associate of Arts degree, and he was considered to be an above average student. When assigned to the program for job-search skills, the patient had established a record for being on time to out-patient treatment programs, was motivated to seek employment, and had good social skills. His limitations were decreased attention span and lack of attention to detail, poor self-image and inability to use public transportation. He was obese, had an unsteady gait, and used an optic scope on his glasses.

To reduce these deficits the patient was assigned to various simulated work groups with the goal of increasing his attention span and endurance. The patient was given a hygiene check list with instructions to improve his personal hygiene. He also received verbal feedback from other patients in his group about his personal hygiene.

The patient learned to use public transportation by memorizing specific bus routes and was accompanied by the assistant who rode the bus with the patient to reinforce his learning. The patient has lost 40 pounds and improved his self-care so that it is appropriate for work in an office. Improvement in appearance contributed to improved self-concept. He learned to pay attention to details and obtained work in a training program as a clerk, a job in which he was able to work a full eight-hour day with lunch and two breaks, indicating increased endurance. The patient does labeling, and the assistant made a template guide so that the patient can affix the press apply labels accurately on envelopes or file folders.

This patient has been on his job over a year, uses public transportation independently to and from work, and reports that he feels like a man again.

CASE DESCRIPTION 2

A number of patients who have been referred to the program cannot seek work because of illness, age or the possibility of losing a pension or disability check if they seek remunerative employment. Therefore, these patients are encouraged to seek volunteer activities as they would a job.

A 54-year-old widow with bi-polar disorder was referred to the program. Although she had worked in a nursing home for ten years, she was unable to return to nursing because of her psychiatric disorder. Each time she reached the point in the job preparation program when it was necessary to have a job interview, she became too "nervous" to go. After re-evaluating her goals and fears related to employment, it was learned that she would lose her only source of income, her husband's pension.

It was then suggested that she consider volunteer work at a Senior Citizen's Center near her home. She could go to the Center without spending money on transportation, which appealed to her because of her fixed income. She was assigned to the Meals on Wheels Program and helps deliver food to homebound residents. The benefits this patient received from participating in this program included increased social interactions, feelings of being needed, and receipt of a free meal each day she volunteered at the Center. The Center put her in contact with several agencies that assisted her in paying her bills, and once every six months she and other volunteers are taken on special event trips, with expenses paid, in appreciation of their service. This patient found part-time volunteer work that was beneficial to her and to the organization she served.

RESULTS

Kramer and Beidel (1982) suggest that additional study be done to compare the SCORE program with other programs for teaching job-search skills to the chronically mentally ill. Although the program at UTMB was not implemented with a research emphasis, a year after implementation seven low level patients with a long unemployment history have obtained employment, and two have obtained volunteer work. One employed member of the group has been promoted in the job he found as a result of the job-search program. Of the 70 patients who have been through the program in two years about one-half have been able to find jobs independently. This certainly validates the usefulness of the SCORE training modules.

CONCLUSION

A program to teach job-search skills was implemented by an assistant on the staff. The program was based on SCORE and, repeated SCORE's success in teaching chronic mentally ill patients how to look for and obtain employment.

REFERENCES

Andersen, A.P. (1985). Work potential evaluation in mental health. *American Journal of Occupational Therapy*, *39*, 659-663.

Clakeley, G.L. (1988). Designing employee enrichment projects. *Occupational Therapy in Health Care*, *5*(2/3), 47-53.

Deacon, S., Dunning, R.E. and Dease, R. (1974). A job clinic for psychotic clients in remission. *American Journal of Occupational Therapy*, *28*, 144-147.

DeMars, P.K. (1975). Training adult retardates for private enterprise. *American Journal of Occupational Therapy*, *29*, 39-42.

Howe, M.C., Weaver, C.T. and Dulay, J. (1981). The development of work oriented day center program. *American Journal of Occupational Therapy*, *35*, 711-718.

Kramer, L.W. (1984). SCORE: Solving community obstacles and restoring employment. *Occupational Therapy in Health Care*, *4*, 1-135.

Kramer, L.W. and Beidel, D.C. (1982). Job seeking skill groups: A review and application to chronic psychiatric population. *Occupational Therapy in Mental Health*, *2*, 37-44.

Puccetti, D. (1988). Supervision of the COTA: Developing a knowledge base and strategy. *Occupational Therapy in Health Care*, *5*, (2/3), 23-35.

Stauffer, D.L. (1986). Predicting successful employment in the community for people with a history of chronic mental illness. *Occupational Therapy in Mental Health*, *6*, 31-49.

Watts, F.N. (1976). Modification of the employment handicaps of psychiatric patients by behavioral method. *American Journal of Occupational Therapy*, *30*, 487-490.

Strategies for Resolution of Intraprofessional Conflict Related to the Role of the Certified Occupational Therapy Assistant

Barbara Forté, BSVE, COTA, ROH

SUMMARY. The certified occupational therapy assistant's role continues to be of concern to our profession. Occupational therapy personnel have identified the same issues, especially role confusion and inadequate supervision, as problems without clear solutions for almost two decades. The author addresses these and other problems and proposes use of de Bono's lateral thinking style for problem analysis and resolution.

INTRODUCTION

More than ever before the occupational therapy profession is confronted with the need to be more externally oriented as its members continue to define and expand the practice of occupational therapy and its particular niche in providing health care services. A void has been created with the transition of registered occupational therapists

---

Barbara Forté is a 1972 graduate of Los Angeles City College Occupational Therapy Assistant program. She was granted an instructor's credential in Health and Physical Care Services and Related Technologies in 1981 and received a Bachelor of Science degree in Vocational Education, with a minor in Human Resource Management from California State University, Long Beach in 1983. Ms. Forté resigned as Director of Program Services for First Step Independent Living, Inc., San Bernardino, CA in October, 1986 and currently is a full-time graduate student in biology at California State University, San Bernardino.

This article appears jointly in *Certified Occupational Therapy Assistants: Opportunities and Challenges* (The Haworth Press, 1988) and *Occupational Therapy in Health Care*, Volume 5, Numbers 2/3 (1988).

(OTR or therapist) from the role of generalists to specialists with a corresponding requirement that they assume different levels of responsibilities. Many therapists have been reluctant to let go of technical skills that were part of their domain of practice prior to recognition of the certified occupational therapy assistant (COTA or assistant). Some of this reluctance arises because the education of therapists has, of necessity, focused on acquisition of clinical knowledge and in the past has not generally included knowledge of and experience in supervision, particularly as both are relevant to the utilization of assistants.

The certified occupational therapy assistant (COTA or assistant) has unique and specialized skills and knowledge. As the technical component of the occupational therapy profession, assistants are able to provide the technical and functional aspects of treatment and rehabilitative processes. The assistant can be an effective, cost-efficient provider of occupational therapy services as demonstrated by productivity studies that document economic benefits associated with effective use of assistants (Dennis, 1988).

Occupational therapy personnel, regardless of level of certification, can no longer afford to adopt a passive stance about intraprofessional conflict over the roles of the therapist and assistant that can only weaken the overall impact of services. When conflict arises or exists, immediate action must be taken to define goals and objectives of both levels of personnel to achieve unified resolution of problems. This paper will address areas of intraprofessional role conflict, alternative approaches to address those conflicts, and strategies for their resolution.

SOURCES OF INTRAPROFESSIONAL CONFLICT

Issues of role confusion for both therapists and assistants and a need for supervision guidelines have been identified as problems for almost two decades (Brooks, 1982). Areas of overlapping skills have abetted the role confusion. Many therapists have been slow or reluctant to let go of technical skills that were in their domain of practice prior to recognition of the assistant level. Gaps in treatment have also been created by the inadvertent deletion of educational content because of the expansion of clinically related knowledge that therapists must acquire to insure minimum levels of competency for practice (Brooks, 1982). Therapists must recognize that they can capitalize on the ability of the assistant to complete the continuum of service delivery.

These global issues continue to resurface, with the American Occupational Therapy Association (AOTA) and state associations actively attempting to address these and other concerns related to the assistant in the practice of occupational therapy. One major attempt to resolve these issues began in 1980 when the AOTA Executive Board established the Certified Occupational Therapy Assistant Task Force. The original task-limited charge to this Task Force was to provide an inventory of perceived COTA needs and to suggest ways in which the state and national organizations could be responsive to these needs. Later, the charge was expanded to include the study of the results of the COTA Task Force's initial actions and to address additional COTA concerns in the areas of education, practice, and professional involvement.

The support and encouragement to COTAs from the occupational therapy profession was evident by the passage of the resolution establishing a COTA Representative to the Representative Assembly in 1983 and by the Executive Board's continuation of the Task Force through 1985. In response to the COTA Task Force's final recommendations, the Representative Assembly established the Certified Occupational Therapy Assistant (COTA) Advisory Committee to the Executive Board of the AOTA in 1986. Its functions are to serve in an advisory capacity to all levels within the profession and to develop and implement strategies to resolve problematic issues. Prior to 1980 and establishment of the COTA Task Force, emphasis was directed toward establishment and recognition of the assistant's role as a generalist whose training stressed the functional aspects of patient treatment. Emphasis now seems to be on ways by which the occupational therapy profession can satisfy perceived needs of assistants.

Why do these same issues continue unresolved even with increasing support from the occupational therapy profession? Has the actual problem been addressed or merely a symptom? It is suggested that an alternative thinking style be used in problem identification and, more importantly, reaching solutions. The logical, rigid approaches which training in occupational therapy produces has actually interfered with the generation of new ideas and alternatives. Edward de Bono labelled this sequential, logical approach as vertical thinking. He proposes use of lateral thinking as a way to increase the number of potential solutions, stating "the vertical thinker is forever classifying things . . . is more interested in seeing on what basis he can pull things apart, the lateral thinkier is more interested in seeing on what basis he can put things together" (de Bono, 1968). Approaching issues from a different perspective may generate solutions that up to now have not been evident.

Skilled occupational therapy personnel who have acquired post-entry level knowledge through experience or formal education are able to apply their task analysis skills to problem analysis. Such analytical skills are vital to the provision of qualitative occupational therapy treatment. Objective analysis of problems, as well as clear expression of the subjective meaning of underlying issues associated with these problems, will allow united efforts among all occupational therapy personnel to resolve intraprofessional conflicts. By establishing clearly defined objectives first, the effect of defensive reactions will be minimized.

Some major areas and specific issues contributing to intraprofessional conflict will now be addressed.

Role Limitations

Role limitations of the assistant level of practice are a recurring area of dissatisfaction reported by assistants. Assistants see the AOTA, statutory regulations, supervisors, and/or job descriptions as limiting their practice and preventing them from utilizing their abilities and higher levels of skills. COTA members of the AOTA are asking that the AOTA establish policies that will broaden the parameters of the assistant's roles, that will establish some form of recognition for those acquiring post-entry level skills, and to respond to complaints of inappropirate salary differences between the assistant and therapist.

While it appears that the problem to be resolved is one of limits of practice, problem analysis will demonstrate that more specific problems are involved. These smaller components, seen as separate issues, make themselves easier to address. But addressing solutions will require that assistants and therapists each accept their own responsibilities as professionals.

There *are* limitations to practice as an assistant, as there are limits to the practice of other roles requiring licensure or certification. These limits are for the protection of consumers, the professional body of knowledge, employers, and licensees. It is unrealistic to expect basic limits to be fundamentally changed. Once this is acknowledged, time and energy can then be directed toward creating ways to meet the needs of individuals while remaining within the prescribed practice limits.

Therefore, the problem is *not* that there are role limits. Instead, the problem stems from the assistants' and therapists' perceptions of stated limits and their meanings. If an assistant sees parameters of practice as the limits, one solution is for peers to give examples of alternative approaches that have been effective in meeting one's career needs. If one avenue is blocked, look for other avenues rather than continuing to run into the blockage. Re-interpret those terms or phrases in licensure or credentialing statements seen as limiting words. Are they stated as practice mandates without flexibility or are other interpretations possible? Or, realize that the AOTA's guidelines are just that and are not mandatory dictates. For example, the "Guide to Classification of Occupational Therapy Personnel" (Schell, 1985) states that a typical responsibility of an intermediate level staff COTA is to assist in modifying treatment plans under supervision of the OTR. The level of supervision is not specifically stated and can be defined by the degree of confidence the COTA has earned from the supervising therapist. The OTR and COTA as a team must decide the appropriate type and degree of treatment modification the COTA may perform and the amount of supervision the COTA requires. No one statement can reflect all levels of experience and areas of practice.

By their own nature guidelines are general directions that are to be interpreted and used by occupational therapy personnel; ultimate decisions, however, are left to individuals. Realize that existing limits and guidelines are for assistants who practice in specific occupational therapy positions. Having a job title of "Certified Occupational Therapy Assistant" is not the only way to use the unique skills and knowledge achieved through one's education. COTAs must separate their abilities from job titles if they wish to explore other career paths. Each assistant must decide whether satisfaction comes from recognition inherent in a job title or from applying what one knows.

Self-Image

The assistant's self-image is interrelated with the degree of role satisfaction or frustration. Role expansion or role change is sought when there is dissonance between job duties and perception of competency level. In developing his motivation-hygiene theory, Herzberg found separate categories of needs. One category merely prevents decline of worker performance, while the category labelled "motivators" increased feelings of personal satisfaction (Herzberg, 1966).

When needs for personal satisfaction are met in a job, improved feelings of self-worth within the work setting occur. It is suggested that motivational theories and knowledge of organizational behavior will improve the supervisory skills of therapists and will foster the development of the assistant based on the individual's needs and abilities. Conversely, therapists' education requires inclusion of supervisory techniques in the entry-level curriculum.

If therapists are unable to be effective as supervisors, their supervisees will lack clear concepts of themselves as assistants. For example, inherent in the role of supervisor is the responsibility for staff development. Assistants will improve their own self-images within their career track if offered opportunities for structured training and development. Once assistants feel they have a way to meet their needs, decisions to act and the power to change then belongs to them. Feelings of anger and frustration are decreased when assistants feel they are in partial control of solutions affecting their lives (Alvarado, 1987).

Changing Roles of Therapists

Therapists are being asked to make the transition from a position as generalist to a more specialized role demanded by the generation of large bodies of interrelated information now used in practice.

Vamberry (1987) notes that this movement involves a shift of methodology for OTRs from a holistic application of knowledge and skills toward specialized application that requires integration of all appropriate resources to reach sound treatment solutions.

As bodies of knowledge expand, application of techniques becomes more specific due to the large amount of information required to insure competency in any given "specialty" area. Unfortunately, such specialization may exclude addressing patients' wellness (Vamberry, 1987). This shift leaves a void in occupational therapy patient care that is best filled by the assistant who applies global, functionally oriented treatment approaches. The assistant, therein, is the critical link in holistic occupational therapy service delivery. Recognition by the COTA of her importance to the fundamental purpose of occupational therapy is vital to improving her professional self-image. Thus one step toward role satisfaction can be achieved. It is also difficult to look at one level of role functions without also considering other associated levels, especially when using lateral thinking to identify problems.

STRATEGIES FOR CONFLICT RESOLUTION

Emphasizing the assistant's role and responsibilities in the scheme of patient treatment is a finite goal to address. Role models can provide peers with specific strategies thus enabling them to envision more choices and to gain more control of their career growth. Emphasizing the two seemingly most obvious paths for career growth, seeking certification as a therapist or leaving the profession, is a disservice to both the person and the profession. There are always alternate approaches to expand job options if one has the courage and energy to pursue them. For the assistant, a shift in viewpoints is required along with an ability to think in terms of skills and knowledge held, and how and where they can be used, rather than to think in terms of job titles.

Career development can be compared to the development of self-identity, both being dynamic processes having identifiable stages. Career maturation is a process that is developmental in nature and relates to identifiable life stages. For instance, an individual must first attain entry level competencies and become comfortable in a career while simultaneously gaining more self-confidence and maturity before desiring to advance within the chosen career. But this career comfort can only be achieved if the emotional maturation has also reached an equivalent level of growth.

Using career maturity assessments can assist COTAs in redefining their individual needs and identifying job components that are important to them in their choice of new career roles. Movement on the continuum of career maturity will result in COTAs clarifying their individual life goals. Becoming aware of the theoretical concepts in the continual development of career paths can be a valuable tool in retention of occupational therapy personnel (Herr, 1979). Therefore, providing information on self-assessment of needs and motivators is a more realistic strategy for finding satisfying career paths and is far more productive than just listing the reasons for assistants leaving the field. Providing alternatives for growth without requiring letting go of those reasons for choosing the technical level of practice gives COTAs practical alternatives. Assistants who have expanded their skills can contribute to the profession that provided these skills by their commitment to share their learning process with peers.

Personal commitment by COTAs to the growth of the profession of occupational therapy and to their own growth as individuals demands that they have knowledge of existing documents guiding both the education and practice of the assistant level. The Practice Division of the AOTA has compiled the *COTA Supervision Guide* which contains significant guidelines and introductory facts related to role delineation, supervision, and classification of occupational therapy personnel, as well as legal parameters of practice by COTAs under Medicare regulations (AOTA, 1986). To avoid blind acceptance of others' interpretations of the issues, collect opinions from many sources. Ask peers, the state COTA liaisons, and members of the COTA Advisory Committee for their interpretations. Read the profession's publications. Realize that the only way to gain information is to actively seek it through as many available resources as possible. Recognize, however, that the type of information received will simply focus on ideas and general concepts and on other's interpretations. Individuals must synthesize information and integrate it for practical application in the world of work as it applies to one's own career expectations and plans. This approach provides hopeful options for growth and function while utilizing the unique abilities that COTAs have acquired.

CONCLUSION

The Certified Occupational Therapy Assistant is one of two levels of personnel certified to provide occupational therapy services to consumers. The assistant possesses a body of knowledge that focuses on the technical and functional aspects of patient treatment. The void being created by the transition of therapists from generalists to specialists can be appropriately filled by the COTA's functional orientation in treatment approaches.

Role limitation is found in all professions and is realistic as a protective mechanism within a discipline for a broad spectrum of reasons but alternative methods for meeting career and personal needs can be identified within role constraints.

For COTAs, the problems related to their roles and responsibilities continue to be addressed without resolution. Exploring alternative approaches to the job and career paths of COTAs by problem analysis and application of lateral thinking as described by de Bono will depersonalize the issues and provide alternative solutions.

Self-image is part of perceived role limits. Human resource management skills will aid supervising personnel in identifying the needs and motivators of supervisees and in developing staff potential.

COTAs must assume responsibility for their own career roles and realize any transition to new career roles involves learning and acquisition of new information unique to those roles. Emphasis on abilities one possesses rather than on the title given to those abilities will aid in resolving perceived limits and decrease intraprofessional discord.

REFERENCES

Alvarado, N. (1987, March). The forgotten skill. *Mensa Bulletin* pp. 10-12.

Brooks, B. (1982). Cota issues: Yesterday, today, and tomorrow. *American Journal of Occupational Therapy, 36*, 567-568.

Cota supervision guide (1986). Rockville, MD: American Occupational Therapy Association, Inc.

de Bono, E. (1968). *New think*. New York: Basic Books.

Dennis, M. (1988). Calculating cost effectiveness with the certified occupational therapy assistant. *Occupational Therapy in Health Care, 5*(2/3), pp. 37-46.

Herr, E.L. & Cramer, S.H. (1979). *Career guidance through the life span: Systematic approaches*. Boston: Little, Brown.

Herzberg, F. (1966). *Work and the nature of man*. New York: World.

Schell, B.A. (1985). *Guide to classification of occupational therapy personnel*. Rockville, MD: American Occupational Therapy Association.

Vamberry, R. (1987, July 29). Occupational therapists—specialists or generalists. *Occupational Therapy Forum*, p. 9.

Mysticism and Skepticism: Obstacles to the Culturalization of the Certified Occupational Therapy Assistant

Terry D. Brittell, COTA, ROH

SUMMARY. This article will identify beliefs and values held by Certified Occupational Therapy Assistants. These beliefs and values differ from those held by the mainstream culture of the occupational therapy profession and have resulted in the evolution of a subculture among certified occupational therapy assistants. This subculture has the potential to become a force that positively or negatively influences its members as well as the occupational therapy profession. The author will propose strategies to resolve some of these differences, to support certified occupational therapy assistants who will accept responsibility for the challenges which confront them and become a positive force within the mainstreasm culture of the occupational therapy profession.

This article will identify factors that have led Certified Occupational Therapy Assistants (COTAs) to develop a subculture within the American Occupational Therapy Association's (AOTA) mainstream culture.

It appears that there are several types of strategies to resolve the barriers to increasing the involvement of COTAs to the professional association. However, one needs to first identify factors that have led

---

Terry D. Brittell is the Stress Management Program Coordinator at Mohawk Valley Psychiatric Center, Utica, NY 13502.

This article appears jointly in *Certified Occupational Therapy Assistants: Opportunities and Challenges* (The Haworth Press, 1988) and *Occupational Therapy in Health Care*, Volume 5, Numbers 2/3 (1988).

to this problem. These are as follows: lack of autonomy, lack of representation, lack of influence on the educational process, lack of input into role delineation studies, lack of marketing, and lack of communication to ensure that the gains that have been made are not lost. These factors have led to development of a COTA subculture because COTAs have not taken action in regard to these factors.

CERTIFIED OCCUPATIONAL THERAPY ASSISTANTS AS A SUBCULTURE

A subculture is a group within the cultural context of a larger group and has social, economic, ethnic or other characteristics that are unique enough to distinguish it from other groups within the larger group (Deal & Kennedy, 1982). COTAs constitute a subculture because they have a set of values, norms, and standards that differ from those of the mainstream culture of the occupational therapy profession. Examples of values and standards held by COTAs as a subculture include career laddering, availability of continuing education opportunities for COTAs who want to continue functioning at the assistant level and provision of programs at state and national conferences geared to the COTA's educational level. Other issues of concern to COTAs include supervision for experienced COTAs who are beyond entry level practice, role delineation beyond entry level practice, practice in psychosocial dysfunction and exclusion from participation in some of the rituals, ceremonies and functions of the mainstream culture of the AOTA. There are also distinct economic differences and demarcations between the defined roles and responsibilities of the certified occupational therapy assistant and the occupational therapist.

Obviously, some issues and concerns of COTAs differ from those of the parent organization, which is a natural and healthy situation. However, when a subculture adopts values that become incompatible with the larger culture, it has the potential of becoming destructive, not only to itself, but to the culture as a whole. On the other hand, when the larger culture excludes members of subgroups from functions, membership roles and activities, the same thing can occur. Are COTAs going to be leaders or victims? Our association's professional ethics dictate responsibility for oneself.

Each COTA should have a sense of personal responsibility for professional involvement.

Mysticism is defined as "vague speculation or belief without foundation; any theory postulating or based on the possibility of direct or intuitive acquisition of ineffable knowledge or power" (Webster, 1981, p. 1497). Many COTAs view AOTA activities and functions as a mystery, as being irrelevant to them and not easily accessible. Some COTAs feel that AOTA is an entity unrelated to their world and are skeptical about having any input that would be accepted by that entity.

Skepticism is defined as "a viewpoint that universally reliable knowledge is unattainable in particular areas of investigation, or an attitude of doubt or disposition toward incredulity in general or in regard to something particular (as a supported fact)" (Webster, 1981, p. 2132). Many COTAs are unable to believe or understand operations of the parent organization or the reasons for those operations. This produces "skeptics," those unwilling to learn to work in systems and who resist involvement in solving the mysteries of their professional association.

DEFINITION OF CULTURE

Culture is defined as "the integrated pattern of human behavior that includes thought, speech, action, and artifacts and its survival depends on man's capacity for learning and transmitting knowledge to succeeding generations" (Webster, 1981, p. 522). All individuals belong to a mainstream culture as well as to subcultures within that mainstream culture, as determined by heritage, education, environment or social status.

Every organization, like a society, has a culture that provides direction to the membership in terms of the norms, values and behaviors to which members are expected to conform. Understanding the culture of the organization in which one is affiliated is critical to the survival of the individual in that organization. Indeed, individuals who deviate from the cultural norms proscribed by the organization may find themselves disenfranchised and subsequently excluded from mainstream participation. Although COTAs have neither been disenfranchised nor dismissed from the occupational therapy profession, their acceptance of the mainstream culture has been thwarted by their attitudes of mysticism and skepticism about assimilation in the profession's culture. Occupational therapy assistants appear to have slipped from the professional mainstream and have become a subculture of the professional organization. The results are a form of segregation which limits growth of COTAs and deprives the AOTA of full membership support for its activities and goals.

COMPONENTS OF CULTURE

Each culture has "heroes" and "heroines." These are the people who serve as the tangible role models to the rest of the organization. Some heroes are natural born leaders, while some are designated or created by organizations. Perceptive, sensitive members of organizations take a direct hand in grooming people to become leaders, recognizing that others will try to emulate their behavior. These achievers, for they are usually high achievers, are known to virtually every member within the organization, and they demonstrate behaviors linked to success.

Rites and rituals are the systematic, programmed routines of day-to-day life within an organization, and they reward the kinds of behaviors that members are expected to exhibit (Deal & Kennedy, 1982). Ceremonies provide visible and strong examples of the actions and behaviors an organization rewards. An organization with a strong culture specifies in detail the rituals its members are expected to follow.

It is important to understand that culture and related belief systems serve as organizational levers for reinforcing behaviors which create strong identities for members. In this context, each COTA should ask questions. How do the beliefs of AOTA members affect my daily work? How are these beliefs communicated from the organization to the membership, to me? How is my performance as a COTA and as a member of the AOTA characterized? The ability to analyze and answer each of these questions demonstrates one's degree of awareness of the occupational therapy professional culture and its member's roles.

BARRIERS TO COTA INVOLVEMENT IN ASSOCIATION ACTIVITIES

Issues that are seen as barriers to involvement of COTAs in association activities, will be identified and discussed in this section as follows.

The assistant frequently perceives association meetings as failing to address COTA concerns, addressing only the interest of the occupational therapist. Because of this, COTAs find it difficult to participate in the affairs of the association when affairs are only tangentially related to their needs.

Cost is a major factor for many in attending national meetings/conferences as they have limited funds for attending, and it is rare that a facility will provide financial aid.

Even though many COTAs are contributing to practice, as well as to the *OT Forum, Advance*, and *OT Weekly*, there is not a monthly vehicle that clearly allows for communication about professional issues or concerns. There is a section in the *Occupational Therapy News* entitled "COTA Share Column"; however few COTAs contribute to this. Not all contributions have to be positive; they can be in forms of rebuttals or personal opinions. Perhaps the name of this column should be changed to "Do COTAs Care?"

Many COTAs feel that they can not represent therapists in association activities, even though those activities may not have anything to do with education or treatment.

COTAs are prohibited from serving as President, Vice-President, or District Chairperson by the Association's, as well as state affiliates' by-laws. Many state affiliates charge the same dues to both COTAs and OTRs, yet COTAs are not given the same privileges. The rationale for equal membership charges is that the COTA member derives the same benefit as the OTR member in services, such as participation in workshops, conferences, and lobbying efforts, and their costs for both are identical.

For COTAs the major premise guiding their actions is that the assistant provides treatment under the supervision of the occupational therapist to enhance the performance of the patient through a program of activities. These activities have been designed by the assistant and the therapist, or by the assistant under the therapist's supervision, to meet the goals set by the therapist according to assessment of the patient's strengths and weaknesses. AOTA's Role Delineation (1981) states that an entry level the COTA may perform tasks, based on skills and knowledges, that reflect basic training and education. However, the role functions of COTAs vary from facility to facility, and too frequently what the COTA does and what is outlined in the role delineation studies are incongruent.

It appears that the action taken by many COTAs in response to current beliefs about their roles within the profession tend to be passive, restrictive, unintrusive or weak. Those COTAs who have become nationally involved function much the same as the professional therapists who serve on commissions, committees, and task forces. The problem is that too few assistants seek such positions.

Thus, COTAs gravitate to a subculture of and somewhat separate from the mainstream culture. Many COTAs have accepted these barriers, much the same as members of groups such as Women's Rights and The Black Caucus. These groups, as well as the COTA group, appear to function autonomously but have little impact or direct involvement in the mainstream of professional activities as a whole.

Washburn (1976), reporting on the perception of a lack of membership involvement in association activities, found from a survey in her state that there were at least three reasons people did not participate in association activities: (1) physical isolation from other members, (2) lack of interest in formal or national meetings and (3) lack of skills needed to manage individual and group issues. AOTA, through its approaches and offerings to members, has responded to many of these concerns in general. However, for the occupational therapy assistant, many of these issues continue to act as barriers to participation in the AOTA and in state associations.

STRATEGIES FOR RESOLUTION OF PROBLEMS

Listed are possible resolutions/strategies to correct existing barriers.

When subgroups do not have full membership benefits, AOTA administrators should recognize and intervene by appointing subculture group members to general committee membership. This intervention process of meshing member roles produces new options in securing organizational goals. It appears that this is not AOTA's fault as it has created the opportunities; however COTAs have not responded readily. Therefore, full representation of the COTA has failed.

Many COTAs obviously are no longer at entry level. Many are very experienced and specialized. Some have positions that would be considered non-traditional. For example, there are COTAs now working independently in diverse areas of practice, acting as consultants or program coordinators in public schools and in wellness programs. Information about such expanded roles must be shared with COTAs, by COTAs and with the membership of the profession.

There is great need for assistants to market their skills and abilities not only to other assistants, but to therapists, to agencies that employ them, to other professionals, and to the consumer. Essentially "marketing" is defined as an aggregate of functions involved in moving services from the provider (therapist) to the consumer (patient) (Webster, 1981, p. 1383). Occupational therapists are proving their value to society. COTAs must demonstrate their value to the profession.

The expanded roles and services of the COTA need to be communicated to supervising therapists. One way in which this can be done is for supervisors in clinics and hospitals to identify and assign occupational therapy assistants who are role models to act as consultants to other occupational therapy assistants. Occupational therapists and occupational therapy assistants who have formed partnership teams should publicize their partnerships at workshops, professional meetings, the "COTA Share Column" and at conferences. Occupational therapy assistants should provide input on their interests and needs for conferences and meeting activities. For example, both OTRs and COTAs would benefit from a workshop and/or from an article on mentoring and/or supervision.

Occupational therapists and assistants, in general, need to communicate their responsibilities with greater clarity to hospital administrators and physicians. Once responsibilities have been identified, a check list of services provided by entry and advanced level assistants can be developed and circulated among occupational therapy staff which would define functions of the assistants according to their experience. However, these might vary from state to state, depending upon trademark and/or licensure regulations.

Occupational therapy supervisors and departments should be attuned to the skills and responsibilities of the occupational therapy assistant. The occupational therapy assistant with advanced skills could be given greater responsibilities in some areas, e.g., quality assurance, special programming and also in some areas of program planning. Certainly COTAs should recognize and demonstrate the cost effectiveness of their contributions to the treatment process. Supervisors should clarify the roles of COTAs within their own facilities and ensure that these role requirements are compatible with state, federal and association standards.

The COTA must assume the role of marketing COTA services to the consumer. The consumer of occupational therapy services is most often the third party payer who needs to know the difference between OTR and COTA services in order to be assured of the most cost effective service. The consumer needs to understand that the OTR assesses and plans treatment and that the COTA is highly capable of implementing some parts of the treatment plan. Defining these expressed areas could be a function of a task group within any given occupational therapy department to determine how this can be accomplished.

The success and survival of the future for COTAs lie in the area of marketing and must be done by COTAs and the professional association. One should not assume others will do it. COTAs must chart their own destiny within the context of their appropriate roles in relation to those of occupational therapists.

An article entitled "Commitment to State Action," by Hershman (1976), discusses several strategies for resolving these concerns. When applied to COTAs, the strategies suggested are to increase communication networks with other COTAs and with official bodies of AOTA, to increase their own continuing education so as to promote interest in functions of the state and national associations, and to provide themselves with the skills for becoming more assertive, thus enabling them to become advocates for themselves and the profession. Hershman's statement, "Put Action In Your Commitment," provides a sound summary.

MATURATION OF COTAs

Certified Occupational Therapy Assistants have been in existence for 27 years and now approach the period of role refinement and participation in professional activities, typical of the adult approaching maturity and seeking a more viable role. COTAs, eager for an intradependent relationship and having many evolving skills, often find that optimum utilization of their knowledge and skills occurs only in limited settings.

OTRs created certified occupational therapy assistants and must now define and expand their own supervisory/consultancy/treatment roles to share responsibilities for proficiency, accountability and increased potential. As demands change, each occupational therapy assistant must be responsible for maintaining his or her competency. Understanding of the COTA's and OTR's respective functions and integration of the appropriate contributions of each in the area of patient care should promote awareness of the potential both have. COTAs and OTRs must have shared and complementary values and services, rather than competing with each other.

CONCLUSION

Given time and experience, COTAs will be able to blend their subculture with the mainstream culture of the profession. This will occur as they assume responsibility for providing greater input at conferences and workshops, increasing their visibility within the profession and in society, and becoming more actively involved in legislative issues, program planning and creation of new roles for themselves. In taking responsibility for themselves and their professional development they will be able to overcome mysticism and skepticism by knowing how to function in a system.

Participation by COTAs in quality assurance and research will become high priority issues which demonstrate their belief in commitment to the field. For example, quality assurance studies are being designed and carried out by assistants, primarily in their own areas. As example of this is the tracking and study of the management of wheelchair equipment maintenance in a facility. Additionally, nearly forty assistants are currently involved in research projects across the country that involve program evaluation and standardization of assessment tools (AOTA Dataline, 1986, p. 17). Some assistants function as research assistants to occupational therapists, gathering data and/or conducting literature reviews for studies.

In conclusion, COTAs must develop the knowledge and skills to market their services, and in so doing, they will establish their value within the mainstream culture and for society in general. "History has amply demonstrated that if we are unable to meet health care demands in our profession, others will do it for us" (Brooks, 1982, p. 566-567). This is as true for the occupational therapy assistant as it is for the occupational therapist.

The future provides opportunities as well as personal and professional growth, and the COTA must choose to seize the opportunities. COTAs must decide whether they are part of a subculture or mainstream culture. The challenge, in the hands of the assistant, is that of developing strategies and implementing plans to become a vital part of the AOTA. The destiny of the COTA can only be charted by active involvement. If COTAs are not willing to commit themselves to active involvement, they must accept the choice of becoming extinct or remaining in a subculture. Once one becomes committed and involved in professional activities, one will be able to resolve the mysteries of the AOTA and skepticism will be reduced as one's values and beliefs do matter. One way to survive is to create and enhance the creative partnerships of the COTA/OTR. In so doing the profession of Occupational Therapy will become a more viable service to the consumer, which is our greatest value to society.

REFERENCES

Adams, N. G. (1981). Ladder to professional certification: The career mobility program. *American Journal of Occupational Therapy, 35*, 328-331.

American Occupational Therapy Association, Inc. (1985). *Occupational therapy manpower: A plan for progress* (Report). Rockville, MD: Author.

American Occupational Therapy Association, Inc. (1981). *Entry-level role delineation for OTRs and COTAs*. Rockville, MD: Author.

Blechert, T. F. & Christensen, M. F. (1986). Intraprofessional relationships and socialization: The maturation process. In S. Ryan (Ed.), *The certified occupational therapy assistant: Roles and responsibilities*. Thorofare, NJ: Slack.

Brittell, T. D. (1987 May). *Charting our course.* Keynote address presented at the meeting of certified occupational therapy assistant state conference, Middletown, NY.

Brooks, B. (1982). Nationally speaking: COTA issues: Yesterday, today and tomorrow. *American Journal of Occupational Therapy, 36*, 567-568.

Deal, T. & Kennedy, A. (1982). *Corporate cultures: The rites and rituals of corporate life*. Reading, MA: Addison-Wesley.

Hershman, G. (1976). Commitment to state action. *American Journal of Occupational Therapy, 30*, 347-349.

Houle, C. (1980). *Continuing learning in the professions*. San Francisco, CA: Jossey-Bass.

Madigan, M. J. (1985). Characteristics of students in occupational therapy educational programs. *American Journal of Occupational Therapy, 39*, 41-48.

Research Information & Evaluation Division (1986). *Dataline* (Report). American Occupational Therapy Association, Inc. Rockville, MD: Author.

Washburn, M. G. (1976). Nationally speaking: A mechanism to share. *American Journal of Occupational Therapy, 30*, 345-346.

Webster's Third New International Dictionary (1981). Springfield, MA: Merriam-Webster, Inc.

Certified Occupational Therapy Assistants: Preparation for Change

Ronna Linroth, COTA
Penny Boulay, COTA

SUMMARY. The intent of this article is to identify changes in our professional environment and address ways in which Certified Occupational Therapy Assistants can prepare for and adapt to change. The emphasis is on individual responsibility for growth and survival.

INTRODUCTION

Much of what is happening within the profession of occupational therapy is due to growth and maturation accompanied by attitudinal and educational changes among its members. Trends such as more entrepreneurial behavior, more "non-traditional" practice, more personnel with graduate degrees, increased emphasis on research

---

Ronna Linroth, Occupational Therapy Department, Multiple Sclerosis Achievement Center, Riverside Medical Center, Minneapolis, MN.

Penny Boulay, Activities Department, Maplewood Care Center, Maplewood, MN.

The authors wish to express appreciation to Minnesota Occupational Therapy personnel who have created a friendly environment for Certified Occupational Therapy Assistants. For being positive role models for Certified Occupational Therapy Assistants in how to prepare and adapt to change, Toné Blechert, COTA, ROH; Sally Ryan, COTA, ROH; and Barb Larson, OTR, ROH, deserve special mention.

This article appears jointly in *Certified Occupational Therapy Assistants: Opportunities and Challenges* (The Haworth Press, 1988) and *Occupational Therapy in Health Care,* Volume 5, Numbers 2/3 (1988).

and specialization, and more stringent documentation of treatment activity are indicative of these changes. In addition, health care legislation and reimbursement patterns are producing substantial alterations in the profession, as seen most prominently in school system practice. These internal and external forces require occupational therapy personnel to move away from a "wait-and-see" approach. Instead, pressure must be applied to secure occupational therapy a place in the market.

The authors feel strongly that Certified Occupational Therapy Assistants (COTAs) are a viable and valuable asset to our profession. COTAs must take full advantage of the opportunities that change brings. Responsibility must be taken for personal growth and COTAs must begin to define their own directions within the context of individual abilities and limitations. As one practices, there is a developmental continuum of skill as one keeps pace with new technologies in order to provide quality services. Adaptation to the changes in one's profession and in one's professional environment demands a life-long pattern of learning.

Elnora M. Gilfoyle, OTR, FAOTA (1986), president of the American Occupational Therapy Association (AOTA), said that in the future COTAs will be functioning more independently in the areas of evaluation, planning, and treatment. It behooves the COTA to take note and begin preparation to acquire or develop skills necessary to successfully confront these practice changes. The issues identified below are presented for consideration by individual COTAs who want to start their own journeys along the continuum of professional development.

ISSUES

Current issues concerning COTAs are identified in "Occupational Therapy Manpower: A Plan For Progress" (AOTA, 1985) and by the authors of this article. Issues to be discussed include the following, data-based management and documentation, cost-effectiveness of employing COTAs, advanced degrees for personnel, specialization, research, declining demand for COTAs in hospitals, work-life patterns, supervision, and job satisfaction.

Data-Based Management and Documentation

More emphasis is being placed on data-based management and documentation in the health care industry because of increasing emphasis on productivity and cost containment for all disciplines (AOTA, 1985). The "Essentials of an Approved Educational Program for the Occupational Therapy Assistant" (AOTA, 1985) require that curriculums provide specific content and experiences in data collection, including structured observation and interviews, history taking, and administration of structured tests. Required management content for the COTA must include aspects of departmental operations, such as scheduling, record keeping, safety, precautions, and maintenance of supplies and equipment, as well as personnel training and supervision of aides, volunteers, and level I OTA students.

Understanding data collection as it pertains to quality assurance is also required in the assistants' educational preparation. COTAs have much to learn about accountability for productivity and cost containment beyond that required in the "Essentials" (AOTA, 1985) to be prepared for data-based management. Documentation is necessary for any health care discipline: third party payment for services is based on documentation.

Documentation is also a determining factor in quality assurance reviews. COTAs *must* learn to document effectively and accurately. AOTA publishes a guide that is helpful if one works in an acute care facility or restorative program entitled, "Occupational Therapy Documentation" (Kuntavanish, 1987). Assistants working in ambulatory care programs may need to address other criteria in record preparation. At any rate, COTAs must produce clear, concise, well-written notes that are void of misspellings and grammatical errors. If individual COTAs lack good writing skills, getting help to improve them is a good place to start a journey towards greater professionalism.

Cost-Effectiveness of Employing COTAs

The bright side of the issue of accountability for productivity and cost-containment is that it is much more cost-effective to employ COTAs to work with and under the supervision of a therapist than it is to employ only Registered Occupational Therapists (OTRs). Most occupational therapists intuitively know this but a good job of documenting and marketing this fact has yet to be done.

Advanced Degrees for Personnel

Figures show a substantial increase in advanced degrees for therapists and baccalaureate degrees for assistants (AOTA, 1985). This seems to be a natural evolution both as the profession matures and society places more value on education. It has been demonstrated in more mature professions and other disciplines that as more people acquire advanced degrees and expand research endeavors, new jobs and professional responsibilities emerge (AOTA, 1985). Educational advancement for COTAs increases the spectrum of their employment possibilities while it also broadens the parameters of their performance in traditional and non-traditional settings.

Many feel the movement toward requiring entry into practice at the graduate level for therapists appears to be a way of strengthening the profession and its services. The effect of this movement on COTAs has not yet been addressed. Therefore, it is time for COTAs to discuss, analyze, and suggest what needs to be done. If, or when, a Master's degree entry-level occurs, the gap in practice between therapists and assistants may further widen: on the other hand, it may help clarify the separate roles within the profession's scope of practice. It may also provide opportunities for growth in COTA roles and responsibilities. Is the next step a baccalaureate degree for COTAs upon entry into the profession? Many factors will influence such a decision but the answer may be in one's assessment of whether or not a COTA role in the profession will be as valid a one as it is today.

Specialization

There is an increased emphasis on specialization (AOTA, 1985). Because of the breadth of the field of occupational therapy, most therapists and assistants tend to specialize in one or two particular areas, usually in an informal way. OTRs have some means for formally recognizing specialization, as with certificates in neurodevelopmental approach to treatment (NDT) or sensory integration (SI).

COTAs, many of whom suffer an identity crisis, must find vehicles to demonstrate their advancing skill levels. For example, COTAs could, through college courses, get a Certificate in Aging, a Bachelor's Degree in Business Administration, or acquire computer proficiency by entering a certificate program in computer science. Recognition of expertise can also come from involvement in state and national associations.

The AOTA maintains a Resource File and Speakers Bureau of COTAs. Submit a vitae and request inclusion in the file system as an advanced-skill COTA. AOTA's Special Interest Section Steering Committee is in the process of developing a plan for occupational therapy personnel to be recognized in specific professional areas. COTAs can create individual plans for developing special skills rather than waiting for other mechanisms to be put in place and can assume responsibility for development of expertise in a specific area of practice. This can be done independently through workshops, selective reading, course work, working or studying with mentors or specialists, or employing a supervisor or consultant to provide direction and guidance.

Research

There is increased emphasis on research within the profession (AOTA, 1985). There does not appear to be any central data collection on the extent of involvement in research by COTAs. A ventured guess is that participation remains minimal. COTAs should begin to think in terms of research interests and team up with a supportive therapist. Various resources are available, and the "National Data Book" (New York Foundation Center, 1987) is an excellent place to identify organizations which might be interested in supporting research projects in one's interest area. AOTA and the American Occupational Therapy Foundation (AOTF) also offer modest research funds. On the other hand, if one has already conducted or participated in research, seek publication of the work. There are now a variety of publications in the professional field which seek manuscripts on such activities.

Declining Demands for COTAs in Hospitals

Demand for therapists is expanding but declining for assistants in hospital settings (AOTA, 1985). To hold a place in the employment market, COTAs need to develop strategies which will enable them to move into new, different, and non-traditional settings. Some alternatives may include such facilities or programs as Adult Day Care, especially for Alzheimer's Disease, or community based programs for the handicapped and elderly that address safety, socialization, activities of daily living, other purposeful activities, and access to established services to maximize their potential for independent living. If the location is right, consider teaming up with a therapist and go "on the road" with occupational therapy to cover rural areas that have previously been underserved.

Work-Life Patterns for COTAs

> It is apparent from statistics that the work-life patterns of COTAs are different from registered occupational therapists. They (COTAs) experience a much higher attrition from the Association and from the workforce, and they exhibit much less job-related mobility than OTRs, thereby potentially reducing employment opportunities. (AOTA, 1985, p.10)
>
> As a consequence (of attrition), the COTA workforce is more likely to be always comprised of assistants who have roughly the same age and experience, and thus the same employment frequency. (AOTA, 1985, p. 28)

The loss of more experienced assistants means that COTAs lose strong leadership and potential mentors or role models who would otherwise be examples of professional growth and a positive COTA image. COTAs with advanced skills do exist. The problem is that they are unrecognized and therefore, are under-utilized as the role models they could be.

Supervision

One cannot discuss COTA issues without addressing the issue of supervision. The amount and frequency of supervision necessary for a COTA to practice occupational therapy varies with each given work situation and with third party payment requirements. Maturity, experience, level of skill in occupational therapy, communication skills, and personality all enter into the establishment of a working relationship as does the facility and type of client seen. This is why there are no cook-book-type definitions of supervision and why written guidelines in specific terms, except for given situations, might be of little value.

When there is conflict in relationships over supervision, it is important to work toward resolution as a team. If the conflict is one of role delineation, "The COTA Supervision Guide" (AOTA, 1986) may be of assistance. Another helpful document is "The Role of Occupational Therapy Personnel" (AOTA, 1978) which states the following:

> The concepts of "occupational performance" and "components of occupational performance" provided the basis for the major distinction between the two categories of occupational therapy practice. (*Performance components* are the learned and/or inherent elements of behavior that permit the planning of the participation in everyday activity. *Occupational performance* is the planning of and participation in everyday activities). COTAs are responsible for evaluating, planning, and implementing intervention programs aimed at improving or maintaining client's functioning in the six occupational performance categories (self-care, work, academics, homemaking, leisure, and play). OTRs are responsible for evaluating, planning and implementing intervention programs aimed at correcting, improving, or maintaining client's occupational performance components (includes the physical, sensory integrative, emotional, interpersonal, and cognitive components) . . . OTRs are expected to be responsible for all tasks performed by COTAs, and both COTAs and OTRs are responsible for evaluation, planning, and intervention. What differs

> is the levels of responsibility and supervision and the objective of the intervention. (p. 1)

Performance components are prerequisite skills to occupational performance. These distinctions are fundamental guides for the functioning and utilization of COTAs.

Job Satisfaction

COTAs must take advantage of this era of change, and there are many ways to increase satisfaction with one's job. Job satisfaction can be increased with an increase in responsibility, autonomy and/or recognition through development of particular expertise and by educational growth. Utilize the intrinsic satisfiers of a position such as opportunities to experience and learn new technologies and techniques, potential for salary increases, or health and educational benefits. Identify and seek extrinsic satisfiers that are available such as presentations at professional conferences. Consider the personal importance of new relationships, sense of confidence and self-esteem gained in performing a job well done, personal and professional growth, respect for and recognition of one's expertise, a sense of independence, a sense of being nurtured and supported, and the self-satisfaction of being able to help or give hope when a client feels helpless or hopeless.

CONCLUSION

Change is an ever-present phenomenon. COTAs who want to be viable assets to their profession, must take responsibility for individual and collective growth and adaptation to the changes occurring now.

Each COTA must begin to define her own direction within the context of personal abilities and limitations. "Educational programs . . . only assist a person in gaining awareness of strengths, limitations, and growth possibilities and then encourage self-directed learning. The motivation to acquire knowledge and ability . . . must be strong within the individual" (Blechert & Christensen, 1986, p. 388). In order to continue progress along the professional growth continuum, COTAs must keep pace with environmental changes. It can be an exciting and rewarding journey.

In conclusion, by preparing for changes now, COTAs will be able to embrace, with both competence and confidence, the challenges and opportunities that the future holds.

REFERENCES

Ad Hoc Committee, American Occupational Therapy Association, Inc. (1987). *Occupational Therapy: Directions for the Future*. AOTA Products, 1383 Piccard Drive, Rockville, MD: American Occupational Therapy Association.

Ad Hoc Committee, American Occupational Therapy Association, Inc. (1985). *Occupational Therapy Manpower: A Plan for Progress*. Rockville, MD: American Occupational Therapy Association.

American Occupational Therapy Association, Inc. (1986). *COTA Supervision Guide*. Rockville, MD: American Occupational Therapy Association.

American Occupational Therapy Association, Inc. (1983). *Essentials and Guidelines of an Approved Educational Program for the Occupational Therapy Assistant*. Rockville, MD: American Occupational Therapy Association.

Blechert, T.F., Christensen, M.F. (1986). Intraprofessional Relationships and Socialization: The Mature Process. In S.E. Ryan (Ed.) *The Certified Occupational Therapy Assistant Roles and Responsibilities* (p. 388). Slack Incorporated, Thorofare, NJ.

Gilfoyle, Elnora M. (June, 1986). *Occupational Therapy Education: Target 2000*. Welcoming Remarks. Presented at the meeting of the American Occupational Therapy Association Commission on Education, Nashville, TN.

Kuntavanish, Anne A. (1987). *Occupational Therapy Documentation: A System to Capture Outcome Data for Quality Assurance and Program Promotion*. Rockville, MD: American Occupational Therapy Association.

New York Foundation Center. (1987). *National Data Book* (10th ed). The New York Foundation Center, 888 7th Avenue, New York, NY.

Some Messages for the COTA on Image, Imagery, and Imagination

Phillip D. Shannon, MA, MPA, OTR, FAOTA

SUMMARY. The purpose of this article is to convey some messages to the COTA with regard to a more active involvement in the profession. The paths that are taken to deliver these messages are the paths of myths and reality as they cross the issue of image, imagery and imagination. If there is an overall message conveyed, it is that COTAs must assume a greater responsibility for their own destiny, and that the reward for accepting this responsibility is inherent in the process of becoming.

FROM THE TOP

A good friend of mine, who happens to be a COTA, accuses me of playing "mind-games." It is true; it is something that I enjoy. Let me provide you with an example.

Once I said to him: "there is evidence to support the probability that within the near future the COTA will become extinct. You (COTAs) can circumvent your extinction, but only if you take charge of your own destiny. Should you choose not to take charge of your own destiny, then at least you ought to prepare for your demise so that you can exit the profession gracefully."

Certainly I did not, and I do not, believe what I said to my friend, but I said it convincingly enough that he did not discount the probability of extinction, although ever so slight. Now my friend is a very

---

Phillip D. Shannon is the Operations Coordinator for Project HOPE's Allied Health Programs in Texas.

This article appears jointly in *Certified Occupational Therapy Assistants: Opportunities and Challenges* (The Haworth Press, 1988) and *Occupational Therapy in Health Care*, Volume 5, Numbers 2/3 (1988).

proactive, creative and productive person who understood my message very well because he shares my concerns for the future of the COTA. Consequently, it was not surprising that he accepted my statement as a challenge to the COTA to become more proactive in the profession.

The messages that follow are presented with the hope that COTAs will not leave their future to chance, but will instead be stimulated to assume a more pivotal role in shaping their own destiny. The paths that are taken to deliver these messages are the paths of myth and reality as they cross the issues of image, imagery and imagination.

ON IMAGE

A few years ago when I was lecturing a new class of occupational therapy assistant students, one student, as I was saying something very profound, of course, rose to her feet and shouted in exasperation, "I just can't take it any longer." Obviously, my lecture came to an abrupt end and I quickly changed roles from educator to therapist in an effort to calm the student and to discover the source of her frustration. And so I said, "my goodness, what is the matter?" The student replied, "occupational therapy is just too (swear word) complex." "You are right," I said, "occupational therapy is an exceedingly complex profession and I would hope that this would challenge you, not discourage you, or discourage any of the other students in the class. Let me assure you that this complexity will seem less so as you progress in the program."

Without elaborating further, the discussion continued after class and the student was able to continue in the program feeling much more confident in her ability to deal with complexity. The purpose in describing this brief scenario is to emphasize the point that anyone who aspires to enter the profession must be prepared to deal with complex concepts and procedures. And why is this warning necessary? Because treating another human being is a complex process that requires the just right blend or mix of specialized knowledge and technical skills, and always, one's very best judgement. If this was not true, then there would be no need for a prescribed period of preparation for becoming an occupational therapy assistant or an occupational therapist. Instead, preparation, as in the case of the occupational therapy aide, would be on-the-job.

Unfortunately, occupational therapy assistants are sometimes perceived as aides, which obviously they are not, nor are they slaves to the occupational therapist. On the contrary, the occupational therapy assistant is a highly trained, highly skilled technician who collaborates with the occupational therapist in the delivery of occupational therapy services to provide comprehensive, balanced programs of treatment.

What should be obvious to all in the profession, which obviously is not all that obvious to some, is that there are differences between the occupational therapy assistant and the occupational therapist. These differences should exist, they do exist, but when they are not apparent something is drastically wrong.

What is wrong when these differences are not apparent stems from a long-standing problem in the profession, the problem or difficulty in clarifying the roles and functions of the occupational therapy assistant and the occupational therapist. These roles and functions simply have not been made explicit, which has blurred the image of the occupational therapy assistant and created differences in perception, that is, how occupational therapy assistants are perceived by others and how they perceive themselves. These problems in perception have caused some occupational therapy assistants to feel somewhat confused or perplexed regarding their professional identity; some feel, and some are, overutilized (performing the work of an occupational therapist); some feel, and some are, underutilized (performing the work of an aide).

It is unlikely that these problems in perception will be resolved in the near future, although a critical first step has been taken with the implementation of the Professional and Technical Role Analysis (PATRA) Project. However, even if the PATRA Project achieves its goal of clarifying the roles and functions of the occupational therapist and occupational therapy assistant (Spelbring, 1987), the image of the occupational therapy assistant will not be altered dramatically without some attention to attitude, or to changing attitudes within and external to the occupational therapy assistant community. Consequently, to reiterate my first message to the COTA, take charge of your future and of changing those attitudes that have an adverse impact on the image of the occupational therapy assistant. If you take no action in this regard, in determining your destiny, then your future will be shaped by default and you will simply have to take "pot-luck."

Taking charge of your future does not mean acting in isolation from the occupational therapist, but in concert with the occupational therapist whose problems with image parallel those of the occupational therapy assistant. Indeed, problems with image have persisted as an incurable plague in the occupational therapy community.

But image, "the concept of someone or something that is held by the public" (American Heritage Dictionary, 1985), has been a particularly nagging problem for the occupational therapy assistant. The source of the problem, some maintain, is nomenclature; if the name is changed from occupational therapy assistant to something else, the problem will be solved.

But, what's in a name? There is nothing special about the name "nurse"; there is nothing very special about the name "doctor." What gives special significance to these names is not the names themselves, but what they have come to mean over time. You can change nurse to "mommie dearest" or "fairy godmother," whichever you prefer, but no matter what the name it is function, not name, that creates the image of a nurse, a doctor, an occupational therapy assistant.

My second message to the occupational therapy assistant is to preserve and promote, not change, the name that is descriptive of the function performed. The occupational therapy assistant assists with the delivery of occupational therapy services. This does not mean that the occupational therapy assistant is an assistant to the occupational therapist. Certainly there are times when an occupational therapy assistant might assist an occupational therapist, just as there are times when an occupational therapist might assist an occupational therapy assistant. However, this is not the rule.

It is the rule in physical therapy. The physical therapist assistant (note the term therapist versus therapy) is an assistant to the physical therapist. Indeed the physical therapist assistant must perform under the direct supervision of the physical therapist. Physical therapist assistants do not enjoy the autonomy, the flexibility that occupational therapy assistants enjoy. Changing occupational therapy assistant to occupational therapy associate, or any other qualifier, will not change image. Furthermore, what has been gained over the years in creating the image of the occupational therapy assistant could be lost if this remedy for the plague is prescribed.

To reiterate, problems with the image of the occupational therapy assistant are not inherent in name but in how those bearing the name perceive themselves and are perceived by others. The strategy for changing these perceptions, for resolving some of the problems with image, is not to change the name but to change the image. The process by which this might be accomplished is the process of imagery.

ON IMAGERY

The process of imagery, which is "producing mental images" (American Heritage Dictionary, 1985) begins in one's own ballpark, at home plate. To get from home plate to first base requires a belief in oneself and in one's capabilities. My third message to the COTA, who wants to get from home plate to first base, is to take pride in being a COTA.

When one does not take pride in who he is, or what he does, acting with confidence and conviction is difficult. It is by one's own behavior that mental images are produced in the minds of others, and to be proud of what one is and of what one does is basic to producing a more positive image of the COTA.

What complicates the issue of taking pride in being a COTA is that many COTAs are repeatedly asked, in one form or another, the following question: "when do you plan to return to school to become an occupational therapist?" Implicit in this question are two messages. The first message conveyed is that the COTA cannot possibly be satisfied with being "just a COTA" all of his or her life. It implies that being "just a COTA," like being "just a homemaker," is not honorable or important work.

The second message conveyed by the question above is that the COTA to whom it is addressed is considered "too smart" to remain "just a COTA," which has two implications. First, that there should not be smart COTAs in the profession; anyone with any "smarts" at all should be an occupational therapist; and second, that most COTAs are basically unintelligent creatures whose actions must be determined and controlled by a superior being.

As glib as these remarks surely seem, the implicit, and usually unintended, messages conveyed when encouraging a COTA to "advance to the therapist level" is what many COTAs hear. Although complimentary on the one hand, on the other hand, pressing a COTA to become an occupational therapist is perceived as devaluing the role of the COTA. Perhaps this is a problem internal to the COTA, perhaps not. Perhaps it is a convenient rationalization for the COTA to resist the pressure to return to school from those who recognize competence and simply want to develop it further. However, this is not the issue.

The issue is: should COTAs stampede their way to professional curriculums in a race to become occupational therapists? Some should, if this is what they truly want. Those who do not want to become occupational therapists should not feel guilty, or be made to feel guilty, when pressed to "advance to the therapist level." Instead, one should reaffirm one's desire to be and to remain an occupational therapy assistant; one should verbalize one's satisfaction and one's pride in being a COTA.

Somebody once said that "OTs want to be PTs; that PTs want to be MDs; and that MDs want to be deities." There is, I suppose, a bit of truth in all humor. However, if I wanted to be a physical therapist I would have enrolled in a physical therapy program. If the occupational therapy assistant wanted, or wants, to be an occupational therapist, he or she had, and still has, that option. To those who wanted, and continue to want, to be an occupational therapy assistant, my fourth message is "why not?" The occupational therapy assistant is a very special participant in promoting and protecting the health and well-being of this nation's citizenry. Certainly the contributions of the occupational therapy assistant in this regard deserve recognition and applause.

Having worked with COTAs throughout most of my professional life, I can appreciate the knowledge and skills that the COTA brings to practice, to education, and to the growth of the profession by participating in the affairs of the Association at all levels. Working side by side as equal partners, one comes to the realization quickly that the COTA has talents that the occupational therapist does not possess. My fifth message to the COTA, in the service of imagery, is to demonstrate these talents and to demonstrate them well. It is by your own behavior, what you do on a day-to-day basis, that others come to know what a COTA is and does. But, like show and tell, not only must you demonstrate your talents well, you must also be a bit less modest in sharing your accomplishments, as in publishing and giving formal and informal presentations, with those significant others with whom you relate. In this way, you will have a greater impact in creating a more positive image of the COTA.

ON IMAGINATION

Imagination, "using the creative power of the mind" (American Heritage Dictionary, 1985), has its rewards in achieving. To achieve is to become, and to become is to realize one's potential. In becoming there is no end point, no final destination. Rather, becoming is like achieving on the installment plan; it persists over a lifetime. The key to becoming is in exercising the imagination.

There are many COTAs who are using the creative power of their minds, who know what it means to become. My sixth message to the COTA is this: follow their example, for they have demonstrated the courage, the stamina, and the imagination to create their own futures. They are the proactive among you, the risk-takers, the achievers, the leaders in the COTA community who have been instrumental in fostering and strengthening the therapist-assistant partnership.

Characteristic of any partnership is that each of the partners is mutually obligated to the other to fulfill certain agreed upon responsibilities. When these responsibilities are explicit, and when they are performed efficiently and effectively in support of some desired or stated goal, it is smooth sailing for the partnership. Sometimes, however, partnerships sail across troubled waters and sometimes creative and innovative solutions are needed to insure that the partnership survives its journey.

My seventh message to the COTA is to assume greater responsibility for steering the partnership to sea and for keeping it afloat when storms threaten on the horizon. This is easier said than done, especially if there is a Captain Hook at the helm.

There are, however, only a small number of Captain Hooks in the profession, and for the most part each of the partners in the delivery of occupational therapy services seeks a dynamic and productive relationship. This relationship can be strengthened by recognizing the special talents that each participant brings to the partnership. Perhaps this is a message of greater significance to the occupational therapist than it is to the occupational therapy assistant.

Nevertheless, if the occupational therapy assistant is to assume greater responsibility for strengthening the partnership, he or she will not succeed if the COTA assumes the passive role of step-child to what is sometimes perceived as the wicked witch. On the contrary, the COTA must project confidence in self and competence in the performance of one's duties. The COTA must become more assertive in expressing his or her beliefs and ideas, to the extent that a true partnership can evolve, characterized by mutual obligation, trust and respect.

I suppose that there might be some occupational therapists who believe that the occupational therapy assistant should be the passive partner in the therapist-assistant relationship, that actions requiring creativity and choice are somehow not within the occupational therapy assistant's capabilities. To assume this position is to deny a fundamental truth that has guided the practice of occupational therapy.

This truth, which is transformed into a principle when treating patients, is that unique to human beings are the capacities for creativity and choice. A prerequisite to exercising creativity and choice, however, is opportunity, which occupational therapy provides in large doses for its patients and claims as one of the guiding principles and unique characteristics of the profession.

If there is a message here for the occupational therapist with regard to the therapist-assistant relationship, there is also one for the COTA. My eighth and final message to the COTA is to allow some time for reflection. From time to time, one needs to reflect upon the past, the present and the future to discover new solutions to old problems and alternative approaches to novel situations. In the absence of reflection, it is difficult to excite the imagination so that it will be sufficiently aroused to generate such questions as "why this" and "what if." But, in the presence of reflection the imagination is unleashed, and it is in exploring the answers to such questions as "why this" and "what if" that the creative power of the mind is permitted to do its best work.

THE BOTTOM LINE

It is an exciting time to be a COTA! Your numbers are increasing at a rapid pace, which gives you greater visibility; you have an Advisory Board that provides input directly to the Executive Board of the AOTA, and to which you can provide input through your Advisory Board; you have greater numbers of COTAs publishing articles and books and chapters in books, as well as greater numbers of occupational therapists publishing materials specifically for the COTA; and there are greater numbers of COTAs delivering presentations at workshops and conferences.

Also, you have more COTAs employed as educators in academic programs for the occupational therapy assistant and for the occupational therapist, and more serving on commissions, committees, and task forces of the Association at the national, state and local levels. You also have greater recognition and greater opportunities to explore, to experiment and to expand your potential.

If there is a movement brewing in the COTA community one can hope that it is a movement toward becoming, for there is so much to be gained by the more active involvement of COTAs in the profession. Perhaps the greatest gain will be that COTAs will not feel the need to be apologetic for who they are, what they do, but that by their more active involvement they will reaffirm their belief in themselves and in their potential.

Surely the time has come when COTAs should be speaking up and speaking out as an affirmation of this belief in themselves. Certainly if I was a COTA, I suppose that I would be among the first to acknowledge this belief; I would be among the first to declare that "I am a COTA, and I'm talking proud!"

REFERENCES

American heritage dictionary (1985). Boston, MA: Houghton Mifflin Company.

Spelbring, L.M. (1987). PATRA project final activities underway. *Occupational Therapy News*, *41*, 5.

PRACTICE WATCH: THINGS TO THINK ABOUT

The *Practice Watch* column has been a vehicle to share items of general concern or topics "on the cutting edge" of practice. It has also been a vehicle for individuals to share ideas and/or experiences that have merit.

This column will be continued, and the Editor invites readers to submit papers that meet the above criteria for review and possible publication. Articles submitted must fulfill the criteria for publication that have been established and that are available upon request from the Editor. In addition, articles submitted for *Practice Watch* may be evaluated on the potential contribution of the article to occupational therapy practice and/or the creativity of the author.

This column will be resumed in the Volume 6, Number 2 1988, issue of *Occupational Therapy in Health Care*.

BOOK REVIEWS

SPINAL CORD INJURY: A GUIDE TO FUNCTIONAL OUTCOMES IN OCCUPATIONAL THERAPY. Edited by Judy P. Hill. *Aspen Publishers, Inc. P.O. Box 990, Frederick, MD 21701, 257 pp., 1986, $39.50.*

This well illustrated manual is a practical guide to the occupational therapy of spinal cord injured (SCI) patients. It offers a comprehensive description of evaluation, program planning, and treatment procedures used at the Rehabilitation Institute of Chicago. An introductory chapter familiarizes the reader with common terminology and with ways to use the guide. The next section focuses on evaluation, goal setting and program planning. The most significant contribution to the SCI knowledge base is contained in a series of chapters detailing specific treatment approaches by the level of injury. These chapters, which make up the bulk of this guide, elucidate and discuss many topics including strengthening methods, deformity control, self-feeding, communication, hygiene and grooming, dressing, bowel and bladder management, bathing, leisure skills training as well as home and community management.

This guide is an excellent resource for the occupational therapy student or the beginning therapist. For experienced clinicians it offers some helpful, easy to find tips to enhance treatment and to solve common problems. This manual's strength lies in its detailed technical descriptions. Quality photography and clear illustrations aid in making this resource a useful, readily accessible tool.

Judy Hill's discussion of strengthening considerations and of deformity control is exceptional. It offers a broad ranging, yet concise, analysis of the relevant factors to be considered in the treatment of the upper extremities of the SCI patient.

Much needed contributions to the occupational therapy literature are found in the chapters discussing bladder and bowel management, the use of electrical environmental aids and special considerations in caring for the pediatric SCI patient. Robin Jones provides a general description of bladder and bowel function and defines the role of the occupational therapist in the management of bladder and bowel care. Janet Bischof contributes an important chapter on the rapidly evolving array of technical aids and electronic equipment presently available to enhance patients' independence in their home and work environments. It includes such devices as call, telephone and environmental control systems, as well as computer adaptations.

Only a few shortcomings were noticed in this guide. Some of the charts were difficult to follow and often attempted to summarize too much information. Additionally, this reader also found the discussion of discharge planning to be unsatisfactory. Although important factors influencing discharge planning were raised, many fundamental issues essential in assuring a smooth transition from the rehabilitation institute to the community were not adequately addressed. It is evident that the same clearly organized, inclusive approach which characterizes earlier sections of this manual was not afforded to the brief and cursory presentation of discharge planning.

All in all, this is an excellent practical guide for the occupational therapist treating the SCI patient. Its broad spectrum of topics, its clear presentation of details, its appealing format, all make it a valuable reference for the clinician.

Michal S. Atkins, OTR
Occupational Therapist
Rancho Los Amigos Medical Center

HAND SPLINTING, PRINCIPLES AND METHODS, 2nd Edition. Elaine Ewing Fess and Cynthia A. Philips. *The C.V. Mosby Co., 11830 Westline Industrial Drive, St. Louis, MO 63146.*

This new edition of Fess' work, dedicated to Hunter, Mackin, and Schneider (parents of the interdisciplinary focus in hand rehabilitation), evidences the increased sophistication of the role of therapists in this area of practice. Retaining the strengths of the first edition (Fess, Gettle, & Strickland, 1981) and adding excellent material, this second edition should provide a resource for therapists at every level of practice.

The contents are organized and presented clearly in six parts plus appendices, bibliography and a new index of splint illustrations. The six parts are: Fundamental Concepts; Principles; Anatomic Sites; Special Situations; Application; and Technique. The strength of the first edition in presenting theory and background material as the basis for specific splint technique has continued and the material in Part One, Fundamental Concepts, has been increased. While Strickland's chapter on the anatomy and kinesiology of the hand has been modified little, he has a completely new chapter on the biological basis of hand splinting from tissue healing (including inflammation and contracture) through joint stiffness and tendon adhesion. The biological rationale for splinting in this chapter adds to the theoretical knowledge vital for the professional working with hand splinting. Additional material on hand assessment (including criteria for valid and reliable instruments) increased the value of this book as a resource or review. The majority of tests mentioned are not described nor specifically referenced (although most seem included in the bibliography) and thus the discussions seem most appropriate to therapists with at least an introductory familiarity with those assessment devices. In contrast, the chapter on classification and nomenclature of splints and components, full of diagrams and photographs, provides an excellent introduction.

The section on Principles (Part Two) was a further content strength of the first edition, and it, too, has added material in this second edition. Mechanical principles are retained essentially unchanged beyond the addition by Thompson (an engineer) of a section on shear stress. While these biomechanical concepts may be unfamiliar to therapists who have not had elementary physics, they are as important a theoretical base as are neurological concepts to our practice. Design, fit and construction principles provide the application of these concepts to these three basic elements of splint fabrication.

Presentations in Part Three, Anatomic Site, and Part Four, Special Situations, describe the application of principles to the fingers, thumb, wrist and forearm in general and for specific diagnostic or functional problems. There is a chapter on the arthritic hand and a chapter on problems ranging from amputation through tendon transfers. A new, although brief, discussion of the controversies in splinting the spastic upper extremity has been added. The chapter on specific problems includes material on integrating a program of splinting with activity to provide the appropriate range of passive, active or resistive exercise.

Part Five, Application, retains material from the first edition that is very useful in learning about common problems and their solutions. A series of splint analyses are presented in two page units with the left page presenting a photo of the incorrect splint described by classification and purpose. The right page includes a drawing of the splint with a description of the clinical problems presented by the errors along with a corrected splint drawing (corrections in red) and the solutions to the problems described. The material is useful for group or individual study and by blocking the right hand side, becomes a self-test of one's analytic ability.

Part Six, Technique, includes an addition of over twenty pages of illustrations for basic splint and component patterns. Each is presented with photographs of a completed splint, of anatomical landmarks marked on the hand or arm, and of a pattern on graph paper background. Accompanying text describes the purposes and lists the important anatomic landmarks. This material, in keeping with the book's philosophy, is aimed more at outlining how to make patterns for the individual than with providing a sheaf of ready-made patterns. A new chapter on plaster casting by Judith Bell-Krotoski presents the concepts of soft tissue remodeling conceived originally by Brand, as the basis for this approach to splinting. She discusses both advantages and disadvantage of plaster and discusses specific applications of the technique not only to the interphalangeal finger joints, but to other structures. Material on negative and positive molds remains essentially unchanged. A brief chapter in the first edition on splinting in a hand surgical practice has been deleted, perhaps because of increased availability of such information by the extensive networking now available through the ASHT.

The first edition of *Hand Splinting* provided a strong scientific basis for the practice of hand splinting with its emphasis upon the biomechanics which form the basis of splinting's effectiveness. Intended as more than a cookbook or compilation of standard patterns, the book reflected the belief that principles of practice must be not only guidelines for techniques, but a grounded basis for the creative approach to problem solving for the individual patient. The second continues and builds on this tradition providing an excellent resource to the profession.

Ruth Zemke, PhD, OTR
Associate Professor
University of Southern California

REHABILITATION PSYCHOLOGY DESK REFERENCE. Edited by Bruce Caplan. *Aspen Publishers, Inc., 1600 Research Boulevard, Rockville, MD 20850, 547 pp., 1987, $42.00.*

The *Rehabilitation Psychology Desk Reference* is a major new resource for professionals concerned with the treatment of rehabilitation patients' psychological and neurobehavioral problems. This comprehensive work presents the latest in research as well as practical information. Clinical procedures, case examples, and outlines of treatment programs provide the reader with proven ways to help patients and families deal with the psychological sequelae that results from a physically disabling disease or injury.

The *Reference Book* is divided into six parts. The first presents information on the conditions that comprise the majority of admissions into rehabilitation centers: spinal cord injury, traumatic head injury, stroke, and chronic pain. The causes, consequences, and treatment of these conditions are discussed with extensive and up-to-date references provided. Part II discusses the psychosocial matrix of the patient, family and staff. This section also includes a chapter presenting reasons and solutions for staff distress and burnout which should be mandatory reading for all health care providers.

Neuropsychology is one of the fastest growing areas of rehabilitation. Part III covers this field in depth. A comprehensive review of assessment techniques and methods is followed by descriptions of programs within hospital-based and private practice settings. The information provided is clearly presented and practical.

A variety of psychological treatment techniques is presented in Part IV of the *Reference Manual*. The social consequences of motor and sensory disability are discussed along with techniques to evaluate and develop the social skills of patients. A social skills training class is outlined which could be effective in helping the disabled cope with the world. Additional chapters in this section discuss the use of biofeedback and video games to improve motor ability, the use of behavior modification in rehabilitation, and the effect of physical disability on sexuality. A realistic research approach for the practitioner is reviewed in the final chapter of this section. Single case experimental design approaches and methodology are presented in a manner easily understood by allied health professionals. The features of this approach, i.e., single case samples, repeated measurement, and generalizability make it significant and practical for the rehabilitation clinician. Specific design strategies and detailed examples provide information that can be easily applied to practice.

The final section provides the reader with an overview of the medical aspects of disabling conditions and clinical pharmacology in rehabilitation. Experienced clinicians will find little information that is new.

The *Rehabilitation Psychology Desk Reference* should be a primary resource manual for both students and practitioners. Including descriptive material as well as guidelines for intervention, this book provides state-of-the-art summaries of the theories and practice of rehabilitation psychology. An emphasis on the effects of psychological conditions on function makes the *Desk Reference* an especially useful tool for the occupational therapist working with physically disabled patients.

Cindy Burt, MS, OTR
Manager, Occupational Therapy Services
University of California at Los Angeles

[illegible] state-of-the-art summaries of the theory and [illegible] of [illegible] pathologies. An emphasis on the effects of psycho[illegible] [illegible] conditions on function makes [illegible] [illegible] [illegible] [illegible] to the occupational therapist working with physically disabled patients.

[illegible], MS, OTR
[illegible] Occupational Therapy Services
University of California, Los Angeles

THOUGHTS ON LEADERSHIP . . .

This section, devoted to leadership, is new to *Occupational Therapy in Health Care*. In this issue Marion W. Crampton and Ruth A. Robinson, who were instrumental in the creation of Occupational Therapy Assistants, will be featured, and their contributions will be discussed. In future issues, other early and outstanding leaders who have made significant contributions to occupational therapy will be introduced.

Certified Occupational Therapy Assistants: Reflections on Their Thirtieth Anniversary

Jerry A. Johnson, EdD, OTR, FAOTA

The year 1988 marks the 30th anniversary of the implementation of the Certified Occupational Therapy Assistant Program in Psychiatry. As this issue of *Occupational Therapy in Health Care* was devoted to the concerns, contributions, and future of Certified Occupational Therapy Assistants (COTAs), it is appropriate to consider the situation which led to the development of this program.

Two registered occupational therapists (OTRs), Ms. Marion W. Crampton and Colonel Ruth A. Robinson, U.S.A. Ret., were interviewed together to discuss their roles in the development and recognition of COTAs. Throughout the interview both Ms. Crampton and Colonel Robinson acknowledged the contributions made by many of their professional colleagues, especially those who served on committees related to this development. The Editor regrets that time and money precluded interviews of at least some of these individuals.

This article, which covers the period through October 1958, will identify some of the qualities and values of Ms. Crampton and Colonel Robinson and will discuss the interrelationship of their personal beliefs and professional motivations, as well as those of their

---

Correspondence may be addressed to Jerry A. Johnson, President, Context, Inc., Denver, CO 80220.

This article appears jointly in *Certified Therapy Assistants: Opportunities and Challenges* (The Haworth Press, 1988) and *Occupational Therapy in Health Care*, Volume 5, Numbers 2/3 (1988).

colleagues, with forces in the social and political climate that contributed to the recognition of the need for occupational therapy support personnel. Their commitment to develop plans for the education and recognition of this level of personnel will also be explored.

Some of the steps involved in the early development of these plans and their adoption by the Board of Management of the American Occupational Therapy Association in 1958 will be discussed briefly. Finally, the reflections of both Ms. Campton and Colonel Robinson on the evolution of COTAs and their present perspectives about the movement will be presented.

Ms. Crampton and Colonel Robinson had different backgrounds and experiences when they became occupational therapists. Ms. Crampton had majored in Spanish at Wellesley College and planned to become a translator. Her studies covered not only the Spanish language but also the literature and customs of the Spanish people. In the opinion of the writer, this desire to become acquainted with another culture was evidence of a love of learning which, combined with a willingness to participate in new experiences, has been characteristic of Ms. Crampton throughout her life. As a professional, it has led her to use many resources and personal contacts to acquire knowledge that she then used to enrich the profession of occupational therapy.

Colonel Robinson, who had the "good fortune" to attend many schools and three high schools, graduated from the Katherine Gibbs School at the time of the depression. She was then employed by a Wall Street bank doing financial research, later, by R. H. Macy's department store handling customer complaints and adjustments and finally as secretary and assistant to a radiologist. This helped her in the development of concepts of management efficiency and cost effectiveness.

When she decided to become an occupational therapist, she felt she should learn as much as possible about the profession prior to a final commitment. She therefore volunteered in the social service department at Massachusetts General Hospital, which she judged to be an objective vantage point. She was nonetheless astonished when, as an affiliating student, she discovered the number of non-occupational therapy tasks students were expected to perform, including painting the walls of a clinic. This was contrary to her ideas on education and personnel utilization.

Throughout the interview, it became quite clear that while it was unstated, both Ms. Crampton and Colonel Robinson had a commitment to serve others and a set of moral and ethical values that provided direction to their lives. Both received their professional education at the Boston School of Occupational Therapy (BSOT) and were influenced by its President, Mrs. Majorie B. Greene, who imbued her students with the belief that their profession was special and that they must become involved and participate in professional activities. For example, "It never occured to us to run for office. If we did, we felt it was an obligation. If elected, it was hard work, but we enjoyed the challenge just as we did when we served on committees."

The personal qualities and experiences of both Ms. Crampton and Colonel Robinson and their beliefs about the innate value of occupational therapy formed (at least in the mind of this writer) the basis for the motivation and courage that enabled them to assume leadership roles and fulfill, in the face of often strong opposition, their commitment to formalize the preparation and recognition of an assistant level of personnel within the occupational therapy profession. The rationale was to maintain and increase occupational therapy personnel.

Ms. Crampton and Colonel Robinson were in practice when the United States of America entered World War II. When the war ended, the value of rehabilitation of servicemen with both mental and physical disabilities had again been demonstrated. The need for occupational therapists and other rehabilitation personnel increased. The demand for programs for special needs groups burgeoned and many new programs were started. Support for these programs came as a result of an increase in the availability of both public and private funds.

During this period, Ms. Crampton worked in a state hospital which, when she started there in 1941, was well staffed with occupational therapists and students, visionary physicians who were committed to improving the care of the mentally ill, and professionals from many other disciplines. During the course of World War II she saw the staff being depleted to meet the needs of the military and personally experienced the results of the shortage of occupational therapists and other professionals and the impact this had on patient care.

Ms. Crampton was confronted with the statewide shortage of occupational therapists in 1952 when she accepted a position as the first occupational therapy supervisor in the central office of the Massachusetts Department of Mental Health (MDMH).

One of her first tasks was to survey all the state institutions for the mentally ill and the mentally retarded. She found that while some OTRs were employed in facilities in Metropolitan Boston, very few were employed in other areas around the state. A small number of persons employed as occupational therapists were graduates of an unaccredited program. In addition, employees who were not occupational therapists could be promoted into occupational therapy positions because there were no educational requirements in the state civil service laws and regulations for several unlicensed health professions. Experience was considered a substitute for education for many years.

Most members of occupational therapy departments knew little, if anything, about programs in other facilities. To counter this isolation, Ms. Crampton initiated meetings of head occupational therapists, following the patterns established by the social work and nursing supervisors. The purpose was to develop more dialogue through monthly meetings which were both administrative and educational in nature. She drew on the resources, knowledge and skills of her professional peers in other disciplines and sought to utilize what she learned to enhance and expand the growth of occupational therapists in the system. As a result of these meetings, regular visits to the occupational therapy departments and the introduction of seminars and workshops for department heads and staff members, it became evident to Ms. Crampton that the non-OTRs had a great contribution to make on the technical level.

Colonel Robinson was employed by the United States Army after five years experience in a sheltered and rehabilitation workshop which offered adjustment to and training in all the skills involved in the garment industry from designing, cutting and assembly to selling and office procedures. In the Army she had the opportunity of working in situations where the utilization of trained technical personnel with professional personnel was basic to successful operation. During the war the Army conducted education programs for occupational therapists. It soon became apparent that neither direct recruitment nor the Army professional education program could produce the personnel needed in increasing numbers.

> A one-month training program for occupational therapy assistants was approved in late 1944. Successful applicants were members of the Women's Army Corps and required to have completed basic military medical training and have a background of teaching plus some knowledge of handicrafts or expert handicraft ability plus high school education and an aptitude for teaching.[1]

Observing the success of the program and the contribution made by its graduates served to confirm Colonel Robinson's belief in the wisdom of the use of nonprofessional personnel.

Ms. Crampton became aware of the seriousness of the national shortage of occupational therapists in 1953 after becoming the Massachusetts Association for Occupational Therapy's representative to the House of Delegates of the American Occupational Therapy Association (AOTA) and then an elected delegate member to the Board of Management. She found that states such as Pennsylvania, Wisconsin, and New York had serious personnel shortages similar to those in Massachusetts and were faced with many of the same problems. It was during this period that she became an increasingly ardent advocate for the recognition and utilization of an assistant level of personnel. At the same time, she served on an AOTA committee, headed by Ms. Florence Stattel, OTR, which was charged to "make recommendations for proposed standards of training, accreditation and recognition of non-registered personnel in the occupational therapy program."[2]

Ultimately, Ms. Crampton and Colonel Robinson, who served as president from October 1955 through October 1958, worked together in the American Occupational Therapy Association and shared their mutual concerns about the shortages of personnel in ways that began to produce results. Colonel Robinson, as vice president of the AOTA, was appointed by Ms. Henrietta McNary,

OTR, then AOTA's president, to co-chair with Ms. Gail Fidler, OTR, the Committee to Plan Implementation of Recognition of Non-Professional Personnel in the Field of Occupational Therapy.[3] Ms. Crampton was appointed chariman of a special committee of the Board after the Board's acceptance of the Robinson-Fidler report in October 1955 and the House of Delegates' acceptance of it through a mail vote by January 1, 1956. The charge to the committee was to continue to work and to provide the framework for the recognition and training of occupational therapy assistants in all fields. The final report of the program in psychiatry was accepted by the Board at its October 1957 meeting. The plan was implemented in October 1958. During this period, Colonel Robinson, a keenly interested ex officio member of the committee, was kept apprised of the progress and championed its work when appropriate and indicated.

As the committees developed their charges, the reactions from the field ranged from anger to expressions such as "We can't even define occupational therapy or agree on the educational preparation of the OTR, so how can we train someone else?" There were other difficult times, and as Ms. Crampton said, "I had to learn that when we met as a committee and worked hard during the day on such controversial issues, it was very important to use the evenings for more pleasurable activities so that we could be revitalized."

When Ms. Crampton proposed developing an inservice program for MDMH department members who had no formal training in occupational therapy, the response of the head occupational therapists was favorable. They viewed it as a means of strengthening their own departments. A MDMH committee of head occupational therapists met regularly over a two-year period to develop a one-month program. The first program was offered in 1957, the second program in 1958 was extended to six weeks and the third program, extended to three months, was the first in the country to be approved by the AOTA and became its pilot program.

After the implementation of the AOTA program for training and recognizing occupational therapy assistants in psychiatry, there was still much work to be done and many issues to be worked through. The first task would be to inform state commissioners of mental health and other appropriate agencies and individuals as well as to notify AOTA members and other appropriate bodies of the national and state occupational therapy associations. One of the biggest tasks of the committee would be the review of applications of non-registered personnel to determine if they met eligibility requirements for certification as an occupational therapy assistant by AOTA under a grandfather clause which would be in existence for three years. Another task would be to survey occupational therapy assistant programs, upon request by application, to determine of they met the satndards for AOTA approval, thus qualifying the graduates for certification in a specialty area. Monitoring the progress of a change of bylaws to include a category for certified occupational therapy assistants and their membership benefits would be an unwritten responsibility. Various other matters such as the certification fee and a directory of COTAs would have to be addressed as well.

Another phase of the implementation would be the completion and approval of the program for assistants in general practice. Nursing homes, in particular, were being regulated to meet standards for reimbursement and greatly needed COTAs with a general practice background. Following this would be the consolidation of the preparation of assistants for all areas of practice. The community college development, aided by federal funds, would have to be examined as occupational therapists, as well as other health professionals, would be wooed to establish programs in this setting, some of which would lead to an associate degree. Federal funds would be sought to support workshops to examine the role and function as well as the supervision of the COTA. Integrating the COTAs into AOTA would have to be strengthened. The establishment of a full-time position for technical service director at AOTA's office would have to be budgeted to administer the markedly increased volume of business engendered by the growth and development of COTA activities. All this is another story and should be reported at a later date.

Ms. Crampton and Colonel Robinson, who remained actively involved in the program for many years therafter, when asked how they felt about their contributions to the creation of what is now the "Certified Occupational Therapy Assistant," immediately acknowledged that they had no regrets. Both would take the same stand, even knowing that they were so committed at the time that rejection of their ideas sometimes felt like personal attacks. They strongly believe that occupational therapy assistants strengthened the occupational therapy profession. They expressed satisfaction in the movement of educational programs into community colleges. Once again, they repeatedly paid tribute to many of their colleagues who assisted or supported their efforts to seek recognition of occupational therapy assistants.

In summary, the reality orientation and keen foresight demonstrated by Ms. Crampton and Colonel Robinson enabled them individually to understand the influence and direction of the social and political forces of the times and to relate those forces to the consequences which an extremely serious shortage of registered occupational therapists had for patient care as well as for the future of the occupational therapy profession.

Ms. Crampton and Colonel Robinson, in the syle of true leadership, went beyond the process of establishing relationships, or connectedness, between disparate factors and problem indentification. In some way, each envisioned the contribution that could be made to society, to the health care system, to patients, and to their profession by the creation of an assistant level of personnel within the occupational therapy profession.

Their belief in the validity of this concept enabled them to continue working with their associates over the long period of development of the education, utilization and recognition of this level of personnel by the AOTA. They helped to fulfill a mission in which we can all take pride.

REFERENCES

1. "The Army Medical Specialist" (1968). Office of the Surgeon General, Department of the Army, Washington, D.C. Library of Congress Catalogue Card #68-60001, Superintendent of Documents, Washington, D.C.

2. American Occupational Therapy Association (1953). Meeting of the Board of Management: New Business 2. *American Journal of Occupational Therapy*, *7*, p. 231.

3. Report of the Committee to Plan Implementation of Recognition of Non-Professional Personnel in the Field of Occupational Therapy (1956). *American Journal of Occupational Therapy*, *10*, p. 27.